The
Primary Care Trust
Handbook

~~~~~ Chair

National Association of Primary Care

Foreword by

Chris Ham

Professor of Health Policy and Management
Director, Health Services Management Centre
University of Birmingham

Radcliffe Medical Press

© 2001 Peter Smith

Radcliffe Medical Press Ltd
18 Marcham Road, Abingdon, Oxon OX14 1AA

British Library Cataloguing in Publication Data

A catalogue record for this book is available from the British Library.

ISBN 1 85775 467 0

Typeset by Action Publishing Technology Ltd, Gloucester
Printed and bound by TJ International Ltd, Padstow, Cornwall

Contents

Foreword

The election of a Labour government in 1997 has resulted in continuity as well as change in health policy. Continuity is most apparent in the maintenance of a separation between purchasers and providers. Change is evident in the abolition of fundholding and its replacement with primary care groups (PCGs). Even more important in terms of a departure from past practice is the opportunity for PCGs to become primary care trusts (PCTs) and in the process to take responsibility for the provision of a wide range of community health services. The prospect this holds out is of the emergence of UK-style managed care organisations that have an incentive to provide what they can and to purchase only those services that lie beyond their competence.

The significance of these developments is that they signal a move towards greater collaboration between GPs and a further reduction in professional isolation. In essence, both PCGs and PCTs are networks of primary care providers in which there will be more opportunity than in the past to compare variations in clinical practices and to exert pressure to achieve improvements in performance. The importance of PCGs and PCTs is that this pressure will come mainly from peers rather than managers or politicians. To be sure, it will take time for peer comparison and peer pressure to be widely accepted in general practice but the inescapable logic of the government's policies is that the days of the 'lone ranger' in primary care are at an end and the future is one in which the medical profession as a whole will carry responsibility for standards and performance in an area. GPs will therefore be expected to practise within the framework of local policies and to justify variations from these policies rather than to see them as evidence that clinical freedom is alive and well.

If greater collaboration between GPs is one consequence of PCGs and PCTS, then increased involvement by doctors in management is another. To this extent, general practice is catching up with developments in hospital medicine where the appointment of consultants as medical and clinical directors is now widely accepted. The lesson from secondary care is that involving doctors in management takes time and has to be supported through programmes of training and development. It is also important to distinguish between the leadership role of doctors and the general management support provided by other staff. Effective PCGs and PCTs are likely to be organisations in which there is both credible medical leadership and strong general management that is sensitive to the distinctive characteristics of medical work. Only in this way will the new primary care organisations overcome the scepticism and even resistance of many GPs and put themselves into a position where they can deliver on their promise.

What then should be expected of PCTs as they take on their new role? If the analogy with managed care organisations is accurate, then it is a safe prediction that priority will be given to the adoption of guidelines and protocols to reduce variations in practice. Already this is happening in relation to prescribing and guidelines are also likely to be adopted to influence the referral of patients to hospitals for tests and specialist appointments. PCTs can also be expected to want to strengthen the provision of primary care itself, both to raise standards for patients and to reduce the inappropriate use of secondary care. Put bluntly, if PCTs can consume their own smoke then they will have to spend less on care provided by other organisations. The clear incentive in these arrangements is for even more services to be delivered in the community as primary care and community health services are integrated and as innovations in technology enable a wider range of treatments to be offered outside specialist settings.

It is only a small step from these developments to the establishment of multispecialty medical groups. Such groups have been difficult to form in the past because it made little clinical or financial sense for consultants to work in primary care units serving small populations. The opportunity created by PCTs delivering care to communities of 100 000 or more is to work closely with specialists whose work is based increasingly outside hospital. Paediatricians, geriatricians and psychiatrists, to name but three groups of specialists, are all in this position and a cogent case can be made for many, perhaps most, of the doctors working in these specialties to align themselves with PCTs in recognition of how services are likely to be delivered in the future. In the process, GPs themselves may be able to develop their own skills by working alongside specialists and learning how to provide care directly. Equally, there is no reason why trained nurses should not relieve GPs of some of their current workload to ensure that the time of doctors is concentrated where it can produce the best results.

One final prediction is that PCTs will encourage self-care on the part of patients and their families. In other words, just as the debate about skill mix and staff substitution will change the division of labour between nurses, GPs and specialists, so too there will be delegation from health workers to patients. The opportunities to promote self-service have not been lost on other sectors like banking and retailing and there is no reason why the NHS should not follow suit. With increased availability of information through the Internet and other sources and with technology creating ever-increasing possibilities for self-care, it is easy to see how patients will become co-workers in the medical enterprise of the future. Not only is such a development the likely outcome of rising public expectations and increasingly consumerist attitudes, but also it is in the interests of PCTs to encourage patients to do more for themselves to reduce the burden on hard-pressed professionals.

To make these points is to underline the radicalism of the government's plans in the long term. While it will take time to ensure that doctors are fully involved in PCGs and PCTs, the potential gains in terms of more integrated and accessible services are considerable. The challenge thrown down to GPs is 'manage yourselves or be managed by others'. Those prepared to take up this challenge may surprise even themselves in what can be achieved when professionals are empowered to bring about change.

This handbook will be an invaluable aid to doctors and their colleagues working in and with the new primary care organisations. In explaining clearly and concisely the requirements, functions and relationships of PCTs, the contributors have provided a practical and authoritative guide that will be useful in supporting this process of change and evolution.

Chris Ham
November 2000

List of contributors

Ian Ayres
General Practitioner
Morden Road Clinic, London

Ruth Chambers
Professor of Health Policy
Staffordshire University

Howard Freeman
General Practitioner
The Tod Practice, Wimbledon

Siân Griffiths
Director of Public Health and Health Policy
Oxfordshire Health Authority

David Lyon
General Practitioner
Castlefields Health Centre, Runcorn

Philip Moore
Chair
Kingston Primary Care Group

Roger O'Brien Hill
Chief Executive
Kingston Primary Care Group

John Oldham
Director
Primary Care Collaborative

Robert Sloane
Formerly, Chief Executive
Andover Community Trust

Rod Smith
General Practitioner
Balmore Park Surgery, Caversham

Peter Smith
Chair
National Association of Primary Care

CHAPTER 1

Introduction to PCTs

Rod Smith and Peter Smith

The NHS Plan launched in July 2000[1] placed PCTs and care trusts squarely at the centre of future developments. PCGs will all be expected to become PCTs. PCTs will at some time be expected to shed their fourth skin and emerge in a fifth stage of development, the care trust.

Although initially met with suspicion, PCTs have become the acceptable face of profession-driven planning. Despite early resistance from GPs, nearly 50% of PCGs applied for trust status for April 2001 and up to 80% were expected by 2002. Despite this apparent enthusiasm, many PCGs will have to go through painful reconfigurations to emerge as PCTs.

Some of the early difficulties arose out of misunderstanding as to the nature of PCTs. Figure 1.1, which shows the direction of travel on the New NHS 'Stairway to Heaven' (rejigged to include care trusts) as indicated in *The New NHS: modern, dependable*[2], appears deceptively simple. But such diagrams belie the huge changes required to scale the different steps. Put simply, PCTs are a completely different animal from PCGs and care trusts are another animal again. There is no evolutionary process between them, no missing link. This is key to the understanding of many of the problems that PCTs raise and the many solutions presented in this book.

Much central guidance has been issued on PCTs covering areas such as HR[3], estates[4] and governance arrangements.[5] This book is not an alternative to those documents. Rather, it attempts to cover the many important, practical make-or-break issues that could not be covered by guidance.

The contributors to this book present real solutions to the many unique issues to be faced in this new stage of NHS development. This chapter sets the scene, including the historical background, the major issues and a brief overview of what PCTs will look like.

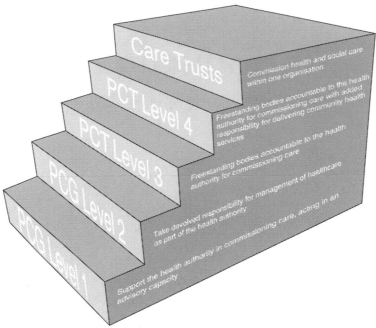

Figure 1.1

Historical background

The New NHS is underpinned by a welfare and support culture that really began in earnest in the late 19th century and bloomed from the beginning of the 20th century, starting with the formation of the Ministry of Health in 1919. The 20th century has been dubbed 'the century of war'. It could be argued that the centralisation inherent within a war effort was exploited to initiate the reforms that led to the NHS Act of 1946, built upon Beveridge's 'five giants of want'.[6] Universality and inclusion were therefore the early drivers.

Since then, other drivers have emerged to produce change and add new dimensions to the delivery of a unique national service.

Cost efficiency

In the 1980s cost control came to the fore in an effort to understand and deal with the spiralling costs of a service about which there were few or no accurate data available. In 1982 a funding review was undertaken by the Secretary of State for Health, Norman Fowler. The conclusion was that a centrally run and centrally funded health service is most effective in controlling costs. Having established that the basis of funding the service was efficient, attempts were made to get to grips with the unruly, uncontrolled NHS by introducing a new management culture.

The Griffiths Report

In 1983, Roy Griffiths, the managing director of Sainsbury's, led an enquiry into NHS management, culminating in a report which concluded:

> *The NHS does not have a profit motive but it is, of course, enormously concerned with control of expenditure … it still lacks any real contin-uous evaluation of its performance against criteria … Rarely are precise management objectives set, there is little measurement of health output; clinical evaluation of particular practices is by no means common and economic evaluation of those practices extremely rare … Whether the NHS is meeting the needs of the patient, and the commu-nity, and can prove that it is doing so, is open to question.*[7]

The concept of general management was introduced to replace the loose consensus management that had been found wanting. However, its success was limited for a variety of reasons. The first was the unusual culture of the NHS, in which clinical freedom was sacred and the nature of the service delivered was therefore largely defined by the profession-als within it. Of equal importance was that in a multibillion pound industry there was little or no accurate information as to what was being spent, where, how, on whom and whether the money spent was produc-ing effective clinical outcomes.

The internal market

Much cynicism surrounds the introduction of the internal market, enshrined in the 1990 NHS and Community Care Act. However, it unequivocally introduced the concept of accountability into the NHS by introducing the purchaser/provider split. It was the internal market that drove the NHS to look at how much it spent and where, because for the first time remuneration was linked to results. If accurate data were not available, a trust or practice would not be paid.

Although the market did not universally address the problems of primary care, it did introduce the concept of involvement of front-line professionals in the business of commissioning. It also introduced within primary care the concept of accountability for clinical behaviour, enshrined within the new Contract and fundholding. The fundholding 'budget', covering referrals, investigations, procedures, drugs, staff and, later, community services, introduced cost awareness into the clinical setting.

In primary care, one of the lasting legacies was the recognition of the importance of good strategic management, an issue that has since been rather overlooked.

Data

Of equal importance was the new part that data began to play. Contracts were usually set on a 'cost per case' or a 'cost and volume' basis. Both required accurate activity data for effective monitoring. For the first time, costs were attributed to measurable events. It was possible to start to understand the true nature of the workings of the NSH and where the money really went.

Quality

In the latter stages of the internal market, contracting for quality began to replace the concept of contracting to achieve savings. With the development of multifunds (fundholding co-operatives) and total purchasing, the notion of strategic contracting for quality within a representative, accountable system took root.

At the same time that many professionals were taking on the role of commissioner, many others became involved in GP commissioning groups, advising health authorities on commissioning.

Despite the criticisms of this era, it produced the ethos and the structures that underpin the structures in the New NHS.

The New NHS drivers

By the mid-1990s, a system had been developed that for the first time had begun to promise real changes in longer term outcomes. However, it had also polarised opinion, producing significant divisions within professions and the public. The perception was also that it had concentrated on secondary care development at the expense of primary care development. Innovators and drivers were motivated to apply their skills to the problems of the NHS. This very success was perceived as accentuating and deepening inequalities in health and healthcare.

Professional issues

The development of the clinical role of nurses in the community in particular meant that the completely GP-centred model was not sustainable. Accountability required that the prescribing and clinical freedom enjoyed by GPs would have to be tempered by other priorities, most notably quality. For instance, evidence of poor practice such as the problems with paediatric cardiac surgery in Bristol hastened the introduction of clinical governance.

Towards the end of the Conservative period of government that produced the internal market, there was an extensive 'listening exercise' that culminated, amongst other things, in the notion of personal medical services. This became the only significant plank of Conservative policy to survive the change in government and has now taken on an immensely important role.

Central expectations

Once the decision had been made to dismantle the internal market, new drivers emerged. For the first time, inequalities in health were to be seriously addressed. The Black Report, published in 1983,[8] had highlighted the real social differences in morbidity and mortality but by the time the Acheson Report was produced in 1998,[9] inequalities had been accentuated further.

Quality

The logical extension of the notion of accountability was that standards needed to be set and systems set up to ensure they were met. This was something of a revolution for the NHS, leading to the adoption of clinical governance and the Commission for Health Improvement (CHI or CHIMP), responsible for ensuring standards are met. This was inevitable, given the inability of the NHS to prevent its own personnel from continuing to indulge in demonstrably dangerous practices as highlighted in the problems with paediatric cardiac surgery in Bristol. The world of absolute clinical freedom ended not with a bang but with a whimper.

Quality was one of the many pillars supporting the New NHS and it underpins many of the new structures. The introduction to NHS bodies of the statutory duty of quality, equal with financial responsibility, was an early marker of the direction of travel.

Rationing

With the burgeoning number of new, expensive therapies appearing, health authorities had adopted different policies regarding the availability of services. This led to the 'postcode lottery', where treatments were not universally available. Central rationing would be introduced to deal with this. Amongst its other roles the National Institute for Clinical Excellence (NICE) would be responsible for taking affordability into account when recommending the adoption or rejection by the NHS of particular therapies.

Consumerism

In a world where resources are restricted, the consumerism driver has been the most difficult to address. Consumerism in the NHS has tended to focus on availability and convenience for those in employment. The cost of such convenience has not been addressed, both in terms of the expensive front-line professionals that deliver the service and the extra stresses placed upon an already disillusioned, overworked and increasingly difficult to retain NHS workforce. All this against a background of low numbers of doctors and nurses by international standards.

One of the unfortunate effects of this emphasis on convenience has been the difficulty for many in accepting the 'patient-centred' NHS. The EU Family Practice Study in 1999[10] emphasised the desire for many of the 'old-fashioned' qualities in the GP role in particular. Society has yet to resolve the dichotomy between desire for a personal service from a GP with a service that is available at all times and is cheap. In its desire for convenience, it may lose some of the real possibilities of a patient-centred service delivered by a personal family doctor or nurse.

Morale

Despite the failings of previous systems, they engendered a feeling of goodwill in the NHS which led to an unrivalled commitment from the workforce. But frequent changes have left morale at a low ebb and raising it will be a huge challenge. If PCTs take on a real support role and deliver a 'bottom-up' approach to meeting the needs of patients and employees, they could achieve the re-engagement of the workforce. The New NHS, through PCTs and care trusts, will need to emulate the success of previous systems in motivating the NHS workforce if it is to achieve lasting change.

The big issues for PCTs

The decision to move to PCT status

The key issue for most PCGs is not whether they should go to trust status but when. There is little advantage in remaining as a PCG for those that are able to make the transition. Management capacity is greatly enhanced by the merger of PCGs with existing trusts to form PCTs. There are also potential efficiencies to be gained by having one organisation managing community services rather than having separate community trusts and PCGs.

In reality, of course, the merger is more complex, as practices functioning as independent contractors for many decades are unlikely to have fully achieved the cultural transition to corporate members of their PCGs.

Once a PCG board has made the decision to seek PCT status it is important that the board makes explicit the advantages that will accrue from that decision, for the public, for their staff and independent contractors. In practice, unless the transition to PCT status coincides with a major service change such as hospital closure, the public is unlikely to oppose the transition. The public is probably more interested in whether the NHS works than the precise details of how it works. NHS staff, on the other hand, are likely to be extremely interested in the transition as many of them will be changing their employer from community trust to PCT and will need to be reassured on the implications.

Decisions will need to be made for some services such as palliative care, specialist hospital outreach nurses such as diabetic community nurses, and specialist community paediatric and respiratory nurses as to whether these are best employed in primary care or acute trusts. Relevant staff will need to be consulted if there is to be a switch in employer. Sometimes employment and clinical governance arrangements may need to be separated, e.g. palliative care consultants may be best placed in a PCT but may wish to share clinical governance arrangements with acute sector-employed oncologists.

GPs and PCTs

The position of GPs in the transition to PCT status is an interesting one. Historically, GPs have been independent contractors and the BMA has fiercely defended their right to remain so. However, younger GPs are probably less committed to independent contractor status than older ones and salaried options are likely to increase with increasing uptake of PMS pilots.

The independent contractor status has led to widely differing styles of practice and levels of service provision within practices. Whilst individual practices have to a variable extent developed a corporate culture, PCGs are in an early stage of bringing all their practices together into a common primary care organisation. Although no single professional group has a veto on the decision to become a PCT, GPs are likely to hold a ballot through their powerful local trade union, the local medical committee. One first-wave PCT chose to ignore the ballot rejection of a move to PCT status.

Fundholding clearly demonstrated that individual GPs control large amounts of resources and can with effort reduce expenditure on unnecessary prescribing or referrals. Whether the effort will be as strong in a PCG moving to trust status in the face of large-scale opposition remains to be seen. The work of PCGs in drawing up a robust case for seeking trust status and spending time and effort on carrying their staff along with them should pay rich dividends when trust status is achieved.

Ultimately a PCT depends on its staff, whose commitment and energy will determine the success or failure of that trust.

Core functions of the PCT

In preparing their case for becoming a PCT the core functions of a PCG need to be considered and the questions answered as to why they would be better delivered as a trust. To reiterate the functions:

- improving the health of and addressing health inequalities of their local community
- developing primary care and community services including reducing variability of services, developing clinical governance and increasing integration of primary and community care services
- advising on or commissioning directly a range of hospital services.

Additionally, level 4 trusts (which most PCGs will seek to become) will subsume the role of community trusts, including the management of community hospitals.

The challenges

PCGs are relatively immature organisations and face a number of key challenges as they move to trust status:

- engagement of stakeholders
- improving healthcare during a period of massive organisational development
- improving both information management in primary care and data for commissioning secondary care
- exploiting the strengths of the merged organisations
- having in place an effective trust board, an executive committee and appropriate management on becoming a PCT
- creating an effective triumvirate of the key appointments of trust chair, executive committee chair and PCT chief executive
- partnership with Social Services
- involving the public.

Engagement of stakeholders

PCGs have had some success in creating effective corporate boards but less success on engaging key stakeholders, their GPs and nurses.[11] Part of the problem has been that very tight funding both for management and improving services has limited improvements in services in practices and the community. PCGs and PCTs need to find ways of involving all stakeholders in the decision-making processes of the PCG/T and using successful service improvements to demonstrate that engagement on committees leads to genuine service improvement. As more funding reaches the service following the 2000 budget, opportunities to achieve demonstrable service improvement should increase.

Improving healthcare during a period of massive organisational development

The workload involved in creating a PCT is huge, particularly where two or more PCGs are merging. A merger of PCGs is much more complex than that of a PCG and parts of a community trust, as practices in most PCGs are not yet really integrated into the corporate structure of their PCG. There is a danger that the organisational development tasks of continuing the momentum of the PCG and merging it into a PCT will consume all the energies of the management team. This could create a vicious circle, where lack of delivery on the PCG/T's main functions, improving the health of the local community, developing primary care and commissioning hospital services, further disengages key stakeholders and, even worse, the public. The PCG will need to ensure that it is not distracted from the key task of improving the NHS.

PMS pilots

One interesting possibility for a PCG to increase stakeholder involvement is for the whole PCG to move to a personal medical services (PMS) pilot.

PMS seems to have engaged GPs and nurses rather more than PCG/Ts, perhaps unsurprisingly as they arose from the bottom-up listening exercise conducted by the previous Conservative government. Many GPs had expressed dissatisfaction with the general medical service (GMS) contract, which incorporates many bureaucratic claims for high-volume activities. These include registration, family planning and maternity claims, the latter subdivided into antenatal visits, delivery, postnatal visits and postnatal examination.

The GMS contract contains little to encourage the delivery of modern, high-quality care. A PCG switching all its practices into a PMS pilot can replace all the anachronistic and time-consuming GMS claims with a contract that encourages high-quality care. Since it is a local contract, it can incorporate the HImP programme, clinical governance, agreed audits, better information management, practice delivery of National Service Frameworks, standards of access to primary care and any other locally agreed contractual agreements.

The PCG gains by aligning their practices to their strategic objectives and the practices gain from a more sensible contract which helps them deliver better healthcare rather than claim their basic pay. In the long term the PCT has a ready-made flexible local contract. Everyone's a winner, including, most importantly, patients.

Improving information management in primary care and for commissioning secondary care

One of the early lessons of clinical governance in primary care is the very variable state of information management in primary care. Many PCGs are IT rich but information management poor. The clinical governance baseline assessment should have identified the quality of Read coding in practices and most PCG/Ts will need to devote considerable training effort to improving consistency of Read coding across their practices and community staff. Without this effort, quality improvement will prove extremely difficult.

A serious casualty of the end of the internal market has been the loss of practice-based information on secondary care. Demand management will be a crucial factor in reducing waiting lists and that will require high-quality information fed back to practices. Benchmarking between practitioners and practices should encourage more considered referrals. Serious commissioning without high-quality information is impossible and the key task of moving work with resources from secondary to primary care, which could increase the efficiency of the NHS, will need good information on what the actual work is that the PCT wishes to move.

Exploiting the strengths of the merged organisations
Practices vary considerably in their management capacity, including their human resource policies. Very small practices, sometimes managed by the GP, may have struggled to keep up with basic legislation such as health and safety. Community trusts will bring expertise in many management areas, which can help PCTs to ensure equity for staff within practices. This will require careful handling as practices remain independent contractors but potentially can deliver major benefits to practices and staff

Having in place an effective trust board, an executive committee and appropriate management on becoming a PCT
For PCTs to hit the ground running and deliver their core agenda, it is vital that trust boards, executive committees and top managers are appointed as early as possible. There is no guarantee that the board and management team that created the PCT will be the same people as those running the PCT, although some are likely to be involved in both processes. Where PCG chief executives are not appointed by the time the PCT is established there is a serious risk of discontinuity. The quality of person required to run a PCT may be on three months' notice from a previous job and timescales are short in the set-up phase of becoming a PCT.

Creating an effective triumvirate of the key appointments of trust chair, executive committee chair and PCT chief executive
The relationship between the three key players is crucial and carries considerable potential for confusion. They will need to put considerable thought into how they can best deliver the objectives of the PCG through their respective roles and relationships.

Partnership with Social Services
Health and social services are inextricably linked and effective partnerships will be crucial in delivering the NHS agenda. The involvement of Social Services departments in the development of PCGs is already creating more effective partnerships. Continuing partnership can further improve the efficiency of the NHS. New Health Act flexibilities, as referred to in *Partnership in Action*,[12] can be used to turn collaboration into real resource and control-sharing partnerships.

Public involvement
This is a key task for PCTs. The consultation period offers opportunities to involve the public and the presence of five lay members on the trust board should ensure some public representation. Interestingly, the exec-

utive committee does not have a lay representative but it is hoped that committees below this will. Lay representation on PCG boards has often proved extremely valuable and a driver for public involvement throughout the organisation; PCT executive committees may wish to co-opt a lay member.

The challenges for PCTs are immense but the potential benefits to be gained by bringing together PCGs with their constituent practices and community trusts into one organisation are greater. PCTs will be able to deliver primary and community care and commission secondary care, offering huge opportunities to improve the NHS by integrating all its services.

Overview of structure and functions of PCTs

The following chapters explore the structure and function of PCTs in detail. This short section provides a brief summary of central guidance on these issues. For greater detail on these structures, see the government website[13] which contains all the circulars. Or, alternatively, obtain the CD-ROM 'Governance arrangements for PCTs', from the Department of Health. It contains all the background documents on PCTs and is a must for all budding PCT-mongers.

PCTs are unlike other NHS trusts in their governance arrangements. They will have a board that will oversee the executive committee, which will be the 'engine room' of the PCT. This unusual arrangement will produce a triumvirate with whom legal responsibility for the trust will lie: the chair of the PCT board, the chair of the executive committee and the chief executive of the PCT.

The make-up of the board

Each PCT will be overseen by a board comprising 11 members:

- a lay chair
- five lay non-executives from the local community (it is expected that non-execs will in future be appointed by the NHS Appointments Commission as referred to in the NHS Plan, not by the Secretary of State)
- the PCT chief executive
- the director of finance
- three clinicians.

Of the latter three professional members:

- at least one must be a GP and
- one a nurse
- one of the three should also be the clinical governance lead
- one should be the executive committee chair.

It will be the responsibility of the professional members of the executive committee to select the two clinicians and the executive committee chair.

The role of the PCT board

The PCT board has three main functions:

- provide strategic oversight and verification of the work of the executive committee
- monitor progress against the HImP
- ensure that the key requirements of public accountability, probity and public involvement are fully met through publicly transparent systems.

Guidance suggests that the board's decision-making processes should:

- take account of public opinion
- prevent conflicts of interest
- ensure compliance with legal frameworks.

The board will be responsible for holding its executive to account on:

- delivery of the vision for which the PCT was established
- compliance with the broad legal framework, NHS law, human rights, etc.
- delivery of the annual accountability agreement (AAA)
- maintaining an effective strategic base.

It will also ensure that:

- the culture and direction of the organisation is in tune with the needs of the local community
- the PCT maintains the best traditions of public service, public accountability and probity, including sustaining external relationships with the public, patients, local government and other partner organisations
- the PCT has clear processes for decision making.

The PCT executive committee

The PCT Executive Committees (Membership) Directions 2000 is required reading and includes the following:

- the executive committee shall have no more than 15 members
- the PCT chief executive (also sits on the board)
- the PCT director of finance (also sits on the board)
- one or two local social services representatives
- professional members, including:
  - one with qualifications and experience in public health
  - medical practitioners (up to seven)
  - nurses (up to seven)
- there must be a majority of professional members
- the chair will be chosen by the executive committee professional members and ratified by the board chair.

The executive committee will be responsible for the day-to-day management of the PCT. This includes developing and initiating service policies, investment plans, priorities and projects to be delivered by the PCT.

Any health professional who provides (or performs) health services to persons for which the proposed PCT would be responsible for commissioning services, is eligible for membership of the PCT executive committee. The PCT may co-opt others to provide advice for dealing with specific local initiatives such as pharmacists, dentists, nurses, other relevant community and practice managers or from other local organisations, e.g. the district council.

Alternative governance arrangements

Prospective PCTs can apply to the Secretary of State to consider alternative governance arrangements. The Nelson PCT, for instance, applied for increased nursing representation. Kingston PCT applied for extra clinician numbers since it was taking on older people's services and services for people with a learning disability.

PCT functions

PCTs will have the same overall functions as PCGs:

- improving (and addressing inequalities in) the health of their community
- developing primary and community health services
- commissioning secondary care services.

Level 3 PCTs will undertake the full range of these functions but will only be able to commission services, not directly provide them. They will be able to employ staff necessary in the commissioning process.

Level 4 PCTs will also be able to provide services, run hospitals and community health services and employ the necessary staff. They will have no direct function to provide general medical services.

NB: A level 3 PCT will not be able to become a level 4 PCT without full public consultation. The idea, therefore, that the PCG will 'try out' PCT status at level 3 is not really sustainable.

It is not deemed appropriate at present for PCTs to take responsibility for certain functions. These include:

- arrangements for public health surveillance (including the prevention and control of communicable diseases)
- the maintenance of cancer registries
- most functions under the Mental Health Act.

Where agreed by all parties locally, PCTs may be able to further support the delivery of GMS to develop primary care locally. Such provisions include the possibility of PCTs employing staff to support GP practices in their delivery of GMS.

Personal medical services

In view of the confusion over PCTs and PMS, the following two paragraphs are quoted in full from the guidance on governance arrangements:

> *PCTs will be able to provide Personal Medical Services (PMS) or to contract with PMS providers. However, for reasons of probity, they will not be able to contract with themselves to provide PMS. Where a PCT wishes to provide or co-provide PMS services they will do so under a contract to their HA.*
>
> *Existing PMS pilots will be able to choose whether they wish their existing contract to remain with the HA or transfer to the PCT. PCTs will be able to develop or support proposals for PMS pilots to be put to the HA. The HA will however continue to be responsible for ensuring*

that the appropriate consultation takes place and for making recommendations as to whether the proposal should proceed.[14]

Conclusion

This chapter has necessarily been brief. Further clarification and advice can be obtained from the National Association of Primary Care, which has led on moving to PCT status. The NAPC may be contacted at: NAPC, Lettsom House, 11 Chandos Street, Cavendish Square, London W1M 9DE. Telephone: 0207 636 7228. email: napc@primarycare.co.uk. Website: http://www.primarycare.co.uk

References

1 DoH (2000) *The NHS Plan: a plan for investment, a plan for reform.* The Stationery Office, London.
2 NHS Executive (1997) *The New NHS: modern, dependable.* Department of Health, London.
3 http://www.doh.gov.uk/pct/pdfs/enclosures/pct3.pdf
4 http://www.doh.gov.uk/pct/pdfs/enclosures/pct3.pdf
5 http://www.doh.gov.uk/pct/pdfs/pctcgver34.pdf
6 Beveridge W (1942) *Social Insurance and Allied Services.* HMSO, London.
7 NHS Management Inquiry (1983) *Letter to the Secretary of State and Recommendations for Action.* DHSS, London.
8 Townsend P and Davidson N (1983) *Inequalities in Health: the Black Report.* Penguin, Harmondsworth.
9 Department of Health (1998) *Independent Inquiry into Inequalities in Health.* Chair: Sir Donald Acheson. The Stationery Office, London.
10 Grol R, Wensing M (1999) Patients' priorities with respect to general practice care: an international comparison. European Task Force on Patient Evaluations of General Practice (EUROPEP). *Fam Pract.* **16**(1): 4–11.
11 Smith J and Regan E *et al.* (2000) *Getting into Their Stride: interim report of a national evaluation of primary care groups.* HSMC, University of Birmingham, Birmingham.
12 Department of Health (2000) *Partnership in Action: new opportunities for joint working between health and social services.* HMSO, London and http://www.doh.gov.uk/pub/docs/doh/partners.pdf
13 http://www.doh.gov.uk
14 http://www.doh.gov.uk/pct/pdfs/pctcgver34.pdf

CHAPTER 2

From PCG to PCT

Howard Freeman

The medical profession more than any other delights in a richness of eponyms. The White Paper *The New NHS: modern, dependable* unwittingly added another to the list – Milburn's arrow. It is alleged that when he first saw the diagram showing the four stages of progression from a level 1 primary care group (PCG) to a level 4 primary care trust (PCT) (*see* p. 2), the then Minister for Health, Alan Milburn, drew an arrow beside it pointing from level 1 to level 4 lest there be any doubt in the minds of either officials or the profession of what the government's aim was. Whether this be true or just the stuff of legends is immaterial as the real direction of travel had been signalled much earlier on.

The New NHS

The White Paper *The New NHS: modern, dependable* was described by many as being an extremely complex document. Its complexity was due to the multiplicity of issues it was trying to address. Within primary care there was undoubtedly a desire to improve overall the quality of GP services. This included some form of guarantee of minimum quality and also to improve or remove the most poorly performing GPs. Partly in order to achieve this and partly to increase financial control over general practice, there was a need to strengthen mainstream NHS management leverage over general practice. This also produced the opportunity to address one of the many nonsenses of the NHS from its inception which was the artificial separation of general practice from the rest of the primary and community medical services. It did not take a great leap of the imagination to see that the same process gave an opportunity to end the other divide in the delivery of services to the community, that between the health service and local authority Social Services. Looking at this in the round also gave the opportunity to begin the debate about the evolution of health service management from appointed health authorities via regional strategic authorities to more representative local operational authorities.

One of the major problems besetting the NHS is clearly that of ever-increasing medical and pharmaceutical innovation at greater cost coupled with the rise in consumer expectation and the demographic shifts of the population. In the last four general elections the British public have voted for parties who have pledged themselves not to overtly increase the tax burden to the individual. Whilst the NHS may be held up by repeated British governments as a jewel, albeit somewhat tarnished, in the crown, it may more realistically be described as an albatross around the neck. The public have been brainwashed for 50 years to expect a universal service free at the point of delivery and few politicians have been brave enough to address this issue. Couple that with the relatively low percentage of gross domestic product that we are locked into spending on the NHS and the issue of money becomes ever more important. The government clearly set out to address this issue within the primary care strategy it envisaged. Not only is primary care completely cash-limited, but it is now responsible for the cash-limited secondary care budget and making all the decisions of priorities and rationing that go with that. Effectively, the shift from PCG to PCT shifts those decisions from health authorities to PCTs.

The pace of change

To deliver this hugely complex changed agenda for general practice, the first step along the path was PCGs, which must be seen as transient organisations before they evolve into the next step of PCTs. At the launch of the White Paper reassuring noises about this being a 10-year change policy were made. The implementation of the overall policy will probably take a decade but the evolution for general practice will be much more rapid. The evolution phase for general practice must be finished before the next phase of the process can be implemented. As ever in the NHS, the political and electoral cycles will interfere with the speed of the process but fewer and fewer now believe that in five years' time any of the 480-odd PCGs will still remain.

The key question must be, is this achievable within the timescale? Whilst it is nice to use the known analogy of the migration of the old directly managed units (DMUs) to NHS trusts in the early 1990s, the analogy does not of course hold good, as these were directly managed NHS organisations and relatively few in number, not disparate groups of independent contractors. Perhaps the better analogy, although one that few dare use these days, is that of the last government's general practice reforms and the development of GP fundholding.

We can draw several lessons from the way that process evolved. There is little doubt that the early waves of fundholders were driven by a number of reasons ranging from a view that the move would improve service delivery for their patients through financial self-interest to political motivation. The numbers in the early years were small but the effect was that of a snowball with the 'me toos' joining the snowball as it got bigger, such that by the end of the scheme the substantial majority of GPs had voluntarily joined it and had it gone on for another two or three years, it is likely nearly all GPs would have ended up within the scheme. The power of the snowball effect must not be underestimated in the migration from PCG to PCT. The danger of it is that many of the later fundholders did not understand exactly what they were doing but just felt driven to do it and many of the problems which occurred towards the end of fundholding arose because of this follow-my-leader herd instinct.

I was personally asked what I believed was the single most important factor necessary in moving from a PCG to a PCT. My response was 'trust'. Trust has to be earned and built up with time and herein lies one of the big dilemmas of the process: is it possible to form the relationships which lead to trust within the period which will be allowed before pressure for migration upwards will be applied? Again it is worth going back to the previous government's reforms to learn the lessons. Out of the GP fundholding scheme evolved two very useful models that we can refer to. These were multifunds and total purchasing projects (TPPs). Both of these evolved voluntarily between groups of GPs who developed a shared vision and from that shared vision began to develop organisations which functioned. Critics will say that they were often like-minded GPs, the groups were not inclusive of everyone and often did not function particularly well. It is easy to be critical. The reality was that new models had voluntarily evolved within general practice and in many places they were inclusive of all and did function well.

If we look at the early waves of PCTs, these pre-existing groupings are proportionately over-represented within them, because they have already developed the relationships necessary to evolve both internally and externally.

What, then, is the minimum period to develop such relationships? This period is clearly going to be different for different groups and will necessarily be longer where there are more problems to overcome. Again drawing on the personal experience I have of working within a TPP and being very involved with other multifunds and TPPs, the minimum period is likely to be three years and may well extend to five years for many groups. The dangers of moving too quickly are obvious. Not having the vast majority of the professionals who will be involved in the PCT committed and signed up to the concept is a recipe for disaster.

The health authorities which seek to push PCGs who are not yet ready for this huge jump from level 2 to trust status will ultimately realise their mistake when they attempt to performance manage the new organisation, which will fail. Equally, there will be dangers in allowing the process to take too long. Going back to the previous reforms, often the groups went through a phase of great innovation and then began to stagnate and lose direction. There is quite clearly an optimum time for the great leap to occur and another test for health authorities will be if they can judge that correctly; history indicates that their ability to sense the temperature of general practice has not in the past been very good.

For the early waves making the transition from PCG to PCT, the process will be ground breaking. It will be easier for later waves, as many of the other players involved will have potentially already gone through the process locally. It will be very important that the learning is not lost and that it does not have to be relearned for successive waves in the local health economies. Again, whilst the need for this is obvious, to achieve it is going to be extremely difficult. The task is rightly being entrusted to individuals yet the mobility of individuals within the NHS is increasing and there is little guarantee that the local remembrancer will be there to impart the learning from an early PCT to a later one.

PCTs and personal medical services (PMS)

There has been much debate about how, or indeed if, the Primary Care Act fits into the present government's agenda on the NHS. Many have suggested it is just an evolutionary dead end, an anachronism which was inherited. Yet the evidence does not support this.

The Primary Care Act was introduced by the last Conservative government in order to deregulate general practice and, to this end, its monopoly role within the provision of primary care. The way it did this was, for the first time, to allow a movement from the previous personal national contract for GPs to a more service-based whole-systems local contract. As part of this, it cleverly removed both the GPs' monopoly right to be the only provider of what became personal medical services to a population and ended their contract-for-life current arrangements by moving them from Part II to Part I of the NHS Act.

The Bill only passed through the House of Commons after the general election had been called and well after the Conservative government had lost its majority in the lower House. It therefore was one of only a few bills which was enacted with the co-operation of the then Labour opposition in the full knowledge that they were about to be the next government. This fact alone is the strongest indicator that certainly at that time Labour felt that within the broad policy of the Bill, there was resonance with their own emerging plans for primary care.

If it is to deliver the agenda envisaged in the NHS White Paper, the ultimate aim of a PCT must be to hold the contracts of all the professionals, both doctors and nurses, who provide the front-line patient care within their organisations. This can only be achieved if all the doctors move into a Primary Care Act pilot situation. It is worth adding that these pilots have a life expectancy, albeit renewable, of three years. Once the status is permanent, the right of the GP to return to Part II of the NHS Act is likely to be lost and effectively the GP's contract is held by a PCT permanently and the length of the contract can be locally determined. There is nothing, though, to say that that contract has to be any more than short to medium term and so effectively you have moved to a situation of franchising general practice.

Of course, within the franchise situation both sides have to negotiate the contractual terms and if GPs are to deliver more within PCTs then they will need to be rewarded if the quality is appropriate. The contract will also be a mechanism to engage the GPs very firmly within a clinical governance framework to ensure that local quality assurance occurs. In such a situation there will be no escape for poorly performing GPs and it can only be a matter of time until the first contracts are ended.

Local contracts with PCTs

Within the Nelson PCG can be seen the test-bed for this situation. All 84 GPs are on locally based contract and the Nelson PCT, based in south west London, will hold that contract. The GPs arrived at this situation through two different routes and 42 have had longer to think this through than the other half. These first 42, who came out of a TPP and were a first-wave PMS pilot, have formed a single partnership. This partnership, the South West London Primary Care Organisation, necessitated change to the Companies Act to enable it to occur, this change being strongly supported by the Department of Health, the British Medical Association and the General Medical Council. Effectively, the Nelson PCT will end up having either one or two partnerships of GPs, all of whom fortunately perform extremely well, who will also be the owners of very well-positioned and high-quality premises which will be the location for services within the communities.

They are already beginning to negotiate the handback of their support services to the trust. The endpoint to this presumably will be that they will purely be contracted to the trust to provide clinical services whilst agreeing with the trust the support that this will require. It is also likely that as the current GPs begin to retire, incoming GPs will not wish to retain the premises and these may end up being sold on either to the trust or to a third party.

If we look at models in southern California and New Zealand where this sort of arrangement begins to occur, then other professionals will end up joining these professional partnerships. Traditionally these other professionals have been community-based hospital outreach specialists such as psychiatrists and geriatricians but as other independent, professionally regulated groups enter the arena there is nothing to stop them joining these partnerships.

These partnerships will further shift the balance from secondary care towards primary care and this could well be even further shifted if the primary care professional partnerships are allowed to hold the budgets themselves for purchasing the secondary care necessary.

At this stage for the PCT life becomes both easier and clearer. Their role is: to reach agreements with the primary care professionals on the level of the service provided in terms of both its breadth and its quality; to monitor this through normal performance management techniques of the health service and via the clinical governance framework; to ensure that where secondary care budgets are devolved to primary care clinicians, they keep within these budgets; to ensure that the support services they are providing for their primary care clinicians are appropriate; to ensure that there is true integration of all the primary care services that they provide. The bonus for them going down the Primary Care Act route is that for the first time they will have true levers to ensure that all doctors and nurses within the trust perform to acceptable standards and are appropriately remunerated. Rather than being a branch line along the evolutionary pathway, the Primary Care Act is actually one of the main stems of the route and will be the mechanism for PCTs of the future to become closer to US-style health maintenance organisations (HMOs).

The future of PCTs

Previously, the shifting of the priorities and rationing decisions from health authorities to PCTs was identified and through the Primary Care Act pilot mechanism the stick-and-carrot approach to the primary care professionals who ultimately make the decisions which cost was also identified. The analogy with HMOs is too close to avoid. There must be caution about too simplistic an analogy, as structural and cultural differences between the UK and the US are great. The NHS is a monopoly provider in the UK and, unlike in the US, an individual cannot shift from one HMO to another. The fact that PCTs will be part of the NHS family and therefore part of a publicly funded and both publicly and politically accountable system is another major difference.

Notwithstanding all this, PCTs will almost certainly evolve into UK equivalents of HMOs. By their very nature, they will be well placed within the NHS family to start looking at the meeting of the publicly funded NHS with private finance. It is likely that they will rapidly move away from the use of Treasury capital for even minor projects but perhaps more important will be the way they move through to managed care and partnerships with the main potential providers of such pathways – the pharmaceutical industry. If one looks a little bit further one could also envisage PCTs and their population evolving into small mutual assurance friendly societies to supplement NHS funding. Over the next decade they will truly be the test-bed of the NHS development.

Conclusion

It is easy to see PCTs as the endpoint of evolution but more realistically it is likely they are but a step on the road. The government has three very different models in place in the constituent parts of Great Britain and no-one can yet be certain which model will prove to be the more robust. The US experience of HMOs has not been good and whilst PCTs will flirt with the model, how it will evolve will take time to clarify. Nevertheless, PCTs will dominate the world of the NHS for the foreseeable future and their success or failure will be crucial to the shape of the NHS in the first half of the 21st century.

CHAPTER 3

The business of trusts

Ian Ayres

Primary care trusts (PCTs) will be free-standing organisations no different in broad governance terms from other existing NHS trusts. They will hold significant budgets for the commissioning and provision of services, employ significant numbers of staff, hold contracts with other NHS organisations and be performance managed by their local health authority. They will perform these roles within tight governance arrangements laid out in guidance from the NHS Executive. Each PCT will have a board with a lay majority and a professionally dominated executive committee. The board will govern and oversee the activities of the PCT and the executive committee will comprise the 'engine house' of the trust, responsible for its operation.

Each PCT will have a chief executive, who will be the accountable officer, and a finance director. Both these posts are identified in guidance as being a requirement of the PCT. Beyond these two full-time officers, trusts will require a range of other managerial and administrative staff to support the board and the executive committee and to deliver the day-to-day operational management of the trust. A key task in the work of establishing a new PCT will be to design the appropriate organisational structure and recruit staff.

The creation of PCTs is a central part of this government's modernisation agenda. Primary care groups (PCGs) and PCTs are seen as being organisations which will rapidly become a real source of power within the NHS and a powerful driver for improving health services. PCTs merge most of the day-to-day operational and commissioning functions of health authorities with the responsibility for providing community health services currently held by community trusts. As increasing numbers of PCGs move to level 4 trust status, so health authorities will be enabled to become the leaner, more strategic organisations envisaged for them in the NHS Executive document *Leadership for Health: the health authority role*.[1]

The future of community trusts as separate discrete organisations is also questionable once large numbers of PCTs take on the provision of community health services. It is possible that, over time, the majority of community trusts will cease to exist as separate organisations, as their functions merge into those of PCTs. Looking ahead several years, one sees a landscape where the provision of day-to-day primary and community health services is through PCTs, overseen by fewer, leaner and more strategic health authorities, with a few providers of specialised community services, such as learning disabilities. From this can be drawn three key issues pertinent to the new PCT's task of designing and recruiting to a new organisation.

- PCTs will be new organisations, significantly different from any other current organisation within the NHS. In establishing them, the temptation to recreate health authorities or community trusts must be avoided.
- PCTs will not start with a clean sheet of paper; they will inherit a legacy of staff and resources that will transfer with the functions they take on. The challenge of PCTs is to build on the wealth of experience and expertise they inherit without recreating the structures of the past.
- In each local health system there needs to be a critical mass of PCTs established and providing a full range of community health services to enable community trusts to be dissolved and health authorities to become fewer, leaner and more strategic. Only then will the savings in management costs that this government requires be achieved. In the transition, when all three types of organisation exist there is likely to be a great deal of overlap and therefore a great deal of pressure on management cost targets.

The rest of this chapter considers the issues that newly appointed PCT chief executives, boards and executives will need to consider when designing and recruiting to the organisation. It does not attempt to define a typical organisational structure or set a template for others to follow. It is likely that PCTs will evolve organisational structures appropriate to their own local needs and situations. At this stage of evolution of PCTs there are likely to be many different models for management and organisational structure. Over time natural selection will probably reduce the number of viable models. However, predicting where we might end up is likely to be neither accurate nor helpful to those struggling with the task of forming a management team and organisation today.

Key tasks

Conventional wisdom states that 'form follows function'. This is intended to imply that we sit down and coolly and carefully consider the functions that a new organisation is there to perform, the skills and expertise required for these functions and from this dispassionate information, design the jobs and roles required to deliver the functions. Laudable though this approach is, it often leads to a position where the organisation that has been designed has jobs and roles that do not fit comfortably with the individuals inherited. However, it is equally true that form can enable function. Organisations that look identical on paper can perform in very different ways in practice. The task of organisational design is never as simple or as straightforward as some management experts would have us believe.

Appraisal of inherited staff

A key task in the early stages of developing a PCT organisation and infrastructure is an honest appraisal of the skills and expertise of the staff that have been transferred into the new organisation. Not just those skills and expertise evident in previous organisations and roles, but those which the individuals are capable of, with development and support. Understanding an individual's true potential is never easy and it becomes even harder when individuals have been through the stresses and traumas of organisational change. Individuals who perform well or have been perceived to perform well in one organisation's structure and context can in another organisation perform badly.

The form of an organisation can affect whether individuals perform to the highest standards. A key task for a newly appointed chief executive, board and executive committee is to understand the true potential of those staff that have transferred into the new organisation.

Developing a shared vision

A newly born baby faced with a barrage of colours, sounds, smells and tastes very rapidly organises these into patterns that become recognised as faces and words and familiar objects. The ability of the human mind to establish patterns and create order out of chaos is one of the wonders of human development. Yet this very strength can, in times of change, become a hindrance to the ability of individuals and organisations to adapt. Individuals and organisations learn from the past and each new experience is interpreted via the experiences that have gone before. In any new situation the elements that are recognised first are those that most closely resemble those of the past. We discard or ignore elements of a new situation which are not recognised and instead we focus on the familiar.

When we approach PCTs and struggle to understand the nature of these new organisations we instinctively interpret them in terms of our prior experience. The risks from this are twofold. First, there is unlikely to be a clear consensus among all members of boards and executive committees as to exactly what a PCT should be. Second, our instincts will be to reinvent those organisations we already know. Another key task for newly appointed chief executives, boards and executive committees is to develop a new and shared vision of what their PCT needs to be.

Understanding PCT functions

PCTs have the same three main functions as PCGs:

- improve the health of the community
- develop primary and community health services
- commission secondary care services.

In terms of the work that PCTs will do to achieve these three objectives, there should be a natural evolution and development from the work that was started as PCGs and the work that healthcare professionals have been undertaking for many years. It is easy to believe that because PCTs represent a natural evolution of the work of PCGs, the organisational structure and forms should similarly evolve. That is not, I believe, the case. Whilst there is a natural evolution of function from PCG to PCT there needs to be a significant revolution in form. PCTs are accountable and responsible for their actions in a way that PCGs are not. PCGs are able to operate within the safe haven of a health authority who can take the difficult decisions regarding resources, budget and performance management. PCTs need to be able to take these decisions on their own.

Another key task for newly appointed chief executives, boards and executive committees is to truly understand the scope and scale of those functions that have been devolved to them. Work needs to be undertaken to ensure understanding of the statutory obligations and responsibilities that the new PCT has taken on. In particular, it is important that the PCT develops a shared understanding with the local health authority and community trust of exactly who is responsible for what.

PCTs exist within different local health systems and the evolution and development of a PCT will be affected by this context. A PCT whose creation will result in the dissolution of a community trust and which will relate to a new-style, lean and strategic health authority has to take on a very wide range of functions and responsibilities in a very short time. It is also likely to inherit significant numbers of health authority and community trust staff to assist it with that work.

A PCT established in a local health system where the health authority will remain substantially in its current form and where the local community trust will remain viable and thriving has to manage a different set of problems. For this latter PCT, the range of functions and responsibilities taken on initially will be smaller and the number of staff inherited from the community trust or the health authority significantly reduced. It is important that the newly appointed chief executive, board and executive committee understand not just the organisational development plans of their own PCT, but also those of other local health service organisations. The ability to deliver successful organisational development for a PCT will depend on how well it fits the organisational development of other local organisations. This will, in turn, impact on the nature of the management team required to support the PCT.

Making sense of the new structures

Although PCTs are being established as local organisations able to respond to the needs of their patients and populations, the organisational structures laid out for them in the guidance are complex. The three key components of this complexity are:

- a **board** with a lay, non-professional majority responsible for the governance and supervision of the PCT
- an **executive committee** with a professional dominance, responsible for the operation of the PCT
- a **chief executive** as accountable officer and management team responsible for delivering the agenda of the PCT.

This tripartite structure of a lay chairman of the board, professional chairman of the executive committee and a chief executive full-time manager will need to work closely together to ensure the complexity is managed successfully. A final key task of the newly appointed chief executive, board and executive committee will be to understand how the roles of each of the three components of the structure fit together. Clear understandings of the respective roles and responsibilities, how they interface and how conflicts are to be managed and resolved will be critical to the successful development of the PCT.

Risks

Before designing and recruiting to the organisation of a PCT, it is worth looking at some of the risks that an organisation faces if it gets things wrong. I am basing this section of the chapter on the work of Bob Sang[2] in helping us to identify a number of the risks we need to manage. His work, which will be more widely disseminated when complete, has identified a number of key risks that we need to manage in the creation of the organisation for PCT. The risks we have identified to date, and we are sure more will emerge over time, are as follows.

The tripartite governance system may not function

There is a risk that the board may become dysfunctional, unable to work in an open and accountable fashion and unable to allow the executive committee and management team to perform their roles successfully. The executive committee may become divergent from the broad body of professionals in the PCT and will be unable to ensure the implementation of the decisions it takes. The management team may become disconnected from the overall agenda for the PCT and will either drown in the detail of operating the trust or become so task focused that it will lose touch with the board and the executive.

PCTs may be unable to develop integrated and managed care systems

They risk being unable to do this if they are unable to recruit or develop the multidisciplinary skill mix required across the whole PCT. PCTs will also need to prove they can deliver services to a high quality in order to retain the confidence of partner organisations in their ability to lead the development of integrated and managed care systems. The re-engineering of care pathways to implement integrated or managed care will require significant improvements to information and IT, which the PCT will need to be able to deliver if it is to be successful. There will also be a need to release resources through the process of re-engineering to invest elsewhere. Failure to achieve this will lead to a failure to deliver the core agenda.

Existing information and performance management systems may not support the needs of a PCT

The current range of information and performance management systems that PCTs will inherit are not geared up to support functions that PCTs are required to provide and a PCT's ability to manage the development of new information and performance management systems will be critical to success.

PCTs may not be able to deliver the public health agenda

PCTs must rapidly develop the ability to implement effective public health interventions, reduce health inequalities and improve the health of the local population. Failure to develop this expertise or to build consensus between the local population, primary and community health service providers and public health professionals will result in the inability of a PCT to deliver its agenda.

PCTs may not be able to address inequalities in primary care

PCTs must be able to retain the full commitment of all practices within the PCT to the developments described in the primary care investment plan and clinical governance framework. Failure to sustain a momentum across the entire constituency of practices and professionals will result in an increase in inequality.

To manage these risks it is important that the core management team for the PCT includes expertise over and above the pure technical confidence of running the PCT. In particular, the management team would need to include the following capabilities.

- **Technical:** the ability to sustain highly effective administrative and IM&T infrastructure that integrates the governance of the PCT with a distributed operations management system.
- **Knowledge management:** the capacity to deliver and synthesise the financial management, logistical and clinical information needs of the PCT leadership, the directly employed service teams and the practice constituency.

- **Sociotechnical:** supporting multiple transitions from a patchwork of legacy systems towards a network of 'end-user' owned systems across the 'whole local system'.
- **Relational:** providing the catalyst and leadership needed <u>across</u> the levels of the PCT 'natural' hierarchy in order to sustain confidence, communications and credibility. Above all, the 'values in practice' of the PCT must be reflected in increasing inclusivity, a demonstrable commitment to equity and a willingness to connect with other systems and processes.

The above analysis of risks and required capabilities leads to the belief that the structure of successful PCTs will be significantly different to that of many existing organisations. PCTs will need to be less like traditional organisational hierarchies with defined roles and relationships and more like open systems with the individuals working within multiprofessional, multiagency teams undertaking defined tasks.

It is likely that the skill mix of the individuals and the skill mix of the team will become the important determinants, rather than the structure itself. Individuals will need to work in a multiplicity of different groups and teams, adopting a project and change management approach to many issues. Such groups of professionals would need to be formed and re-formed over time, to tackle those issues which are high priority at any given time.

Make or buy

Another area of key consideration for a PCT creating its management organisation is to think through those tasks that it must do and those which may be better performed in partnership with others. PCTs have a great deal of freedom to determine which services they provide themselves and which they enter into collegiate arrangements with others to provide. There is a great deal of encouragement from the NHS Executive for PCTs to think through the most effective and efficient ways for them to deliver their functions. Clearly, it would be suboptimal if all 481 of the current PCGs became PCTs, each developing their own capability to provide a full range of corporate and headquarters functions.

PCTs need to be small and focused organisations if they are to be responsive to local need and they need to share non-core functions with others to ensure the value-for-money benefits of scale. All or part of the following services may be better provided on a supra-PCT basis.

- Operational human resources, including management of the relationships with joint staff unions.
- Estates, maintenance and development.
- Capital projects management.
- IM&T.
- Finance, including book-keeping and payment functions, internal and external audit functions.
- Procurement.
- Communications and public relations.

One PCT or other NHS trust could take on the provision of these services for the whole local health system, establish a corporate services agency for the provision of these services to local NHS organisations or even enter private/public partnerships and subcontract the provision of these services to the private sector.

The decision as to whether a PCT ought to provide a particular function itself or enter other arrangements depends on how critical that core function is to the success of the PCT and whether other organisations have the capability to take it on successfully.

It would be a key consideration for the newly appointed chief executive, board and executive committee to determine which corporate functions they must provide for themselves and which are best provided by working in partnership with other organisations.

Four more considerations

In developing their thinking about the appropriate management structure for a PCT, the newly appointed chief executive, board and executive committee must bear in mind another four key issues.

- PCTs have major clinical governance and organisational development agendas to pursue in the early years of their existence. The development of the management team must be linked to both these issues. The management team must be an integral part of the organisational development work and able to fully support this work across the rest of the organisation. Similar linkages will exist with the clinical governance agenda.
- Traditionally, IM&T has been an add-on for the NHS, a tool which professionals use to assist them to undertake their work. In the future this needs to change. IM&T has the potential to allow health service organisations to completely re-engineer the way they operate. Internet and wireless technologies, the increasing integration of voice and data

systems and the NHS information strategy's priority to develop an electronic health record mean that as the NHS embraces these new technologies, the way in which its professionals work can be significantly altered. The PCT core management team will need to understand the opportunities offered by new technologies and work with the whole PCT to bring about the changes that the technology will allow.

• The dominance of professionals on the executive committee of a PCT places clinical professionals at the heart of decisions that bring together financial and clinical imperatives, often pulling in opposing directions. The PCT core management team will need to be able to work with professionals and manage the structure of debate and decision making, so that this potential clash of the sacred (medicine) and the profane (money) is sensitively managed. The integrity of clinical professionals needs to be maintained whilst the PCT overall achieves its financial objectives: a challenge similar to that of 'walking on water'.

• The government has laid out the development of PCGs and PCTs as part of a 10-year agenda to modernise the NHS. By implication, therefore, the initial establishment of PCTs is the start of a period of significant and continued change and development. The PCT chief executive, board, executive committee and management team will need to be able to manage significant and continuous change. It is likely that as PCTs are established and developed there will be mergers of PCTs, integration of PCT functions with the social care functions of local boroughs and the relocation of a number of traditional secondary care specialties into PCTs (for example, geriatrics and dermatology). PCTs face the dilemma of recruiting a management team that can deliver the statutory obligations and functions of a PCT but is also able to support a process of continuous change and development. Thus it is not just the initial skills and expertise of individuals within the management team that will be critical to its success but their potential to develop and grow over time. Continuous professional development will be as important for the management team of the PCT as it will be for the clinicians and professionals involved.

Conclusion

In summary, then, the challenges facing the newly appointed chief executive, board and executive committee of a PCT as they design and recruit to a core management team are many and complex. For those who become trusts first, there will be no models to copy and the temptation will be to replicate the past. As argued above, PCTs need to be quite different from the organisations that exist at present. The best aspects of the current organisations need to be built on, but there are also many ways in which the current models are inappropriate for the role that PCTs have to play in the modernising agenda. The difficulty is knowing which is which.

I have attempted to describe above some of the issues that the newly appointed chief executive, board and executive committee will need to consider in deciding how to design a management team and to recruit to it but finally, success may depend less on getting the structure right than on recruiting the right individuals and developing them to the best of their potential.

References

1 NHSE (1999) *Leadership for Health: the health authority role.* HMSO, London.
2 Sang B (2000) *PCTs: building core capacity.* NHS Executive, London.

CHAPTER 4

Primary care development

Philip Moore

Never before!

Never before has the development of primary care been given the focus and priority that it receives under primary care organisations. Never before have the resources to develop primary care been gathered into a single unified pot – the unified budget. Never before have all the elements of expenditure in primary care been enumerated in a single document – the primary care investment plan. Never before have all the professionals and staff in primary care had the opportunity to belong to a single organisation – the primary care trust.

This is arguably the central platform of the government's plans for PCTs: to develop primary care into something 'better' that will enable it to address health needs for the 21st century. Whatever else happens, it is clear that general practice and primary care as we know it will change, though how much the professionals involved have truly grasped this is variable. Those who have grasped it tend to be branded pessimists, fatalists or collaborators with the government against the profession.

The reality may well be that we are facing one of the greatest opportunities to take what we value most in primary care and build it into a new vehicle for delivery, securing a quality service for years to come. The alternative may be to bury our heads and carry on as if the reforms did not exist. Failing to tackle the issues and build a future for ourselves may end up as a spectator sport in which we are passive witnesses to the demise of the jewel of the NHS.

Never again?

So, will the professions meet this challenge? Will a willingness to think laterally around the hurdles win the day over entrenchment? Will primary care face and answer the question, 'What do we want primary care to look like in 10 years time?' Will a PCT dare to be different from other NHS trusts? Otherwise the development of primary care will remain a poor relative, constantly begging from its glamorous rich uncle in secondary care.

PCT status has not been universally welcomed. Many GPs fear for their independent contractor status but the elements that are pulled together in a PCT provide an ideal vehicle for the development of primary care. It allows a substantially larger management base to support primary care. It unifies the budgets from which primary care may fund its development. It allows the hospital and community health services (HCHS) budget into the same pot with the possibility of viring to primary care to support the provision of appropriate services in the community.

It has been said that 'heroes reflect the paradigm'. If the media are to be believed, the heroes of modern medicine are mainly the high-tech, cutting edge (in every sense!), high-cost and low-volume aspects of healthcare. Primary care now needs its own heroes but the concept of leadership is not usually welcomed in general practice or indeed in the professions at large.

A leader has been defined as someone who is able to lead others where they would not naturally wish to go. Could it be that PCTs will perform the role of such heroes? It is entirely possible that PMS pilots may provide the safety needed to persuade primary care to follow, particularly where they work closely aligned to PCTs.

And such an opportunity may not present itself again for many years to come. *Carpe diem!*

Divergent squint or broad vision?

Narrow-minded PCTs will never develop a broad vision. If you cannot dream a little you should not be falling asleep in board meetings! This is one role the board cannot abdicate without destroying any chance of making the most of the opportunities presented by PCT status. But many find it difficult to be presented with a blank piece of paper and asked to dream.

So how can it be done?

Using what you've got

There is a larger pool of knowledge in the board members than most people realise. In the GPs, community and practice nurses, Social Services, lay and NED members resides a vast reservoir of local information. The difficulty is that much of this is subconscious: it has been picked up not through systematic study but by living and/or working in the area for many years. It is accessed without conscious thought on almost every working day. It plays a subliminal part in most clinical decision making. And it is not easy to marshal into logical format from cold.

Mapping

A useful mechanism to help unlock this is 'mapping' what people know. On a large rough outline of the PCT area, board members can begin to mark factors that are known about the local community: estates, schools, industry, recreation, clinics, shopping areas, where mental health problems seem to concentrate, where street drugs are easily available. The list grows the more everyone gets into the exercise.

The next stage is to ask how the provision of care matches the population distribution and the needs that have been identified by this simple exercise. It is relatively easy to map existing provision alongside the mapping exercise already done. By the time this is done, it may be that 'gaps' will show up.

Then comes a tricky question. At this stage some will want to opt out, saying that it is pointless as it departs from reality and could never be achieved. But try asking yourselves, 'How would we design primary care from scratch to meet the needs of our population as we have just identified them?' If you can hold through and come up with ideas that are not influenced simply by what exists and the feasibility of changing them (a depressing thought at the best of times) the results may surprise you. Of course, it is unlikely that you will be able to implement all the suggestions, but often concepts arise that will be adaptable in some way to the system you have been lumbered with.

Thinking partnership, thinking systems

An important part of this process is to think wider than GPs! Partnership working is the watchword of PCTs and the reforms have to encompass the professionals who are part of the PHCT and Social Services and the voluntary sector and the private sector and ...

The process described is not the only one available but it does serve to illustrate two important aspects that need to be in place if PCTs are to develop primary care. The first is having a vision; not each individual having a part of the vision (what might just be referred to as a divergent squint, where eventually one image is suppressed) but a *shared vision* that has the breadth of everyone's contribution. The second is learning to think in systems rather than purely around your particular piece of the jigsaw. The skill of most primary care practitioners is to focus down on the individual and on the detail. They need to learn to stand back and see the overview. What has been described here allows them to concentrate on the familiar detail and then to stand back and see (literally, visually on the mapping done) the overview. Seeing an overview that has input from such a variety of viewpoints will encourage *systems thinking* – seeing how all the elements interrelate and operate together.

A starting point

Some idea of the current state of primary care in the area is vital. Without it there can be no understanding of the starting point for any developmental process. But it is possible to invest a great deal of time, energy and resources in gathering some of this kind of information so are there sources of data already available to a PCT?

Clinical governance baseline audit

Whilst this audit is primarily aimed at understanding the capability of practices to engage in clinical governance and education, there will be information of value to inform primary care development. This will vary from PCT to PCT. Use what is there!

The health authority (HA)

Large amounts of intelligence are gathered and stored by health authorities. Generally they will be very willing to help PCTs in the process of primary care development by aggregating and presenting data in a way that is useful. Ask them what can be provided. It is likely to include:

- data on primary care premises including space and facilities
- hours of opening and out-of-hours cover
- staff numbers, whole-time equivalents and turnover
- nursing numbers, whole-time equivalents, grades and turnover
- GP workforce profile including ages (and hence future retirement profiles)
- list size trends and demography; turnover of patients
- achievement of items of service (e.g. night visit rates) and targets (cervical smears and vaccinations)
- approval for child health checks and minor surgery

- prescribing behaviour
- the history of usage of primary care development funding
- patient surveys

The Public Health Department

The director of public health publishes annual reports that are a mine of information about the community. Departments are usually only too ready to help PCTs in producing additional information specific to their particular needs.

Primary care

There is often a large amount of untapped resource in the data contained on GP clinical systems. It is admittedly somewhat haphazard in some cases but presents a potentially useful source that is almost invariably underused. Some input may be necessary to help practices extract useful reports but the results will often be worth the effort. With an eye to the future, it is prudent to make sure that all incentive schemes pay out only for data that are computerised.

Community health councils (CHCs)

The NHS Plan proposed the abolition of CHCs and their replacement with a patient advocate system and local authority scrutiny. At present, CHCs participate in regular practice visits with the HA to inspect primary care premises. Visits are also made to community trust premises, some of which will be part of a PCT. They are closely in touch with the public. Any new system should achieve similar results.

Acute and community trusts

Local hospital and community staff are likely to have perspectives on primary care that are difficult to acquire when working in primary care. Asking secondary care about their opinions may be more revealing than you expect. You will need to make a judgement about its objectivity and accuracy!

The Benchmarking Club

This organisation runs a primary care indicator project that has national and, in some cases, PCT-level data on a variety of measures. This is very useful for providing comparisons with your own local situation. The data include:

- demography, numbers of patient removals and allocations
- number of partners and female GPs, age of GPs, percentage of GPs with MRCGP, postgraduate training provision
- whole-time equivalent staff numbers, number of practice nurses, attached CPNs, onsite physiotherapy
- surgery times, disabled access, patient participation, local charters, access to female GP
- computerisation, websites, use of pathology IT links
- prescribing behaviour, availability of prescribing advice to practices
- approval for minor surgery and child health checks
- rate of inadequate smears, breast screening coverage, night visit rates.

The club can be emailed for further information on swatvoi@aol.com

The above represents a selection of existing data that is relatively easy to access. It is important to beware of being too complicated. Keep the starting point simple. Use the information to identify a few quick wins and a few high-profile gains. Do not forget that the local politics of primary care development remains a factor whether we like it or not!

A plan

Strategic planning is a prime responsibility of any board. A plan is a bridge between what exists and what you want, and addresses how you will achieve the change. As already mentioned, strategic planning is not a process that necessarily comes naturally to primary care professionals. Help, though, is at hand in the form of the *primary care investment plan* (PCIP). It is perhaps surprising that the PCIP represents the first time that all the cash-limited elements of spending in primary care have been drawn together in a single document. These monies are part of the *unified budget* and are the major source of developmental work. The PCIP therefore provides a helpful vehicle for planning.

The PCIP:

- describes how existing and additional GMS expenditure will be used
- serves as a planning and development tool for primary care
- focuses on quality and how to improve it
- is based on the local HImP, which includes national priorities
- links with partners, such as trusts and Social Services, for the integration of strategies. This is especially important where there are broken boundaries, i.e. the PCT is included in more than one local authority or health authority area.

It can helpfully lay out the principles which govern the planning process, for example:

- to improve the health of the population of the PCT: working with all the stakeholders to develop the local HImP to improve and protect the health of the population
- to improve the infrastructure of primary care: working with practices to modernise premises, improve facilities and develop information technology so as to offer a more appropriate and efficient environment in which to deliver patient care
- through clinical governance, to improve the quality of primary care: by the implementation of new working practices, implementation of appropriate and effective treatment, devolving responsibility to nurses. This will be achieved through incentivising good practice in a culture that supports training and development
- to offer a seamless service between primary, community and social care: to develop partnerships with community and Social Services to ensure that patient care is co-ordinated and delivered efficiently as well as cost effectively throughout the whole episode of need
- to ensure that adequate secondary care services are commissioned to meet the needs of the population: to develop partnerships and care pathways with the secondary care providers to ensure that efficient and clearly defined transfer of responsibility is maintained.

Chapters

The plan must then detail chapter by chapter the areas of primary care that are to be targeted for development. The plan covers at least three years so it is vital that the work on vision and systems thinking has been carried out before it is written. Chapters are likely to include the following, each one addressing how the unified budget will be used to achieve the development. Obviously, the final content will depend on precisely what has been identified locally as the priorities for development.

- The vision of the PCT.
- How partnerships with other organisations are being developed.
- Communication with stakeholders and involvement of the public; communication will be a fundamental key and merits a full communications policy.
- Some summary of the current situation, including demographic trends, health needs and inequalities.
- Quality and standards: how they will be set, improved and monitored and how incentive schemes (prescribing, clinical governance and HCHS) will contribute to quality.
- Prescribing.
- Details of how the local HImP targets will be met by the PCT.
- Information management and technology: current status, usage and plans for development.
- Workforce planning.
- Premises: quality and plans for development.
- Local development schemes: what services are appropriate, economic and efficient to provide in a primary care setting; how the transfer of the service and funding from secondary care is planned.
- Training and supervision: practice and professional development plans.

Cost pressures

Finally, the plan must address the cost pressures being experienced by primary care. Those involved in commissioning are well used to the annual cycle of cost pressures presented by the trusts. To date, the equivalent in primary care has been largely overlooked. The PCIP is an ideal vehicle to detail these and act as an indicator of where investment may be needed. Examples may include:

- new, expensive drugs, e.g. olanzapine
- implementation of a national service framework, e.g. coronary heart disease and use of statins
- shift of work to primary care, e.g. early discharges, anticoagulation monitoring.

Some pitfalls for the unwary

Structures

Primary care development is not first and foremost about structures. However, if a PCT does not make it obvious through its structure that it is designed to support primary care, it will start at a disadvantage. The whole management structure needs to be designed to provide support for the smaller organisations upon which it relies to deliver services. Not only must it happen but also it must be perceived to have happened! If no-one notices you've supported them, you haven't!

Bullshit detectors

The best of us, the most aggressively anti-management-speak of us can be prone to jargon. Worse, we can make some awful errors of judgement at times. An essential part of any development plan is to have a team whose role is to deliberately sniff out and remove unnecessary and inaccessible jargon and to check the plan for stupidity and obfuscation. People one PCG chief executive refers to as 'bullshit detectors'. Ignore it and tread in the consequences.

Monitoring

Planning is only of use if you know how far you have progressed. It is essential to know where you are at any point. The stakeholders need to know or they become discouraged. The HA needs to know or it becomes nervous. The PCT management need to know to ensure they achieve their performance-related pay. You cannot escape the duty to monitor progress against the plan. It stands to reason, then, that the plan should include milestones and timescales.

Commissioning for dislocations

It is all too easy to lose the connection between commissioning and what is happening in primary care. Unless the link is made consciously and deliberately maintained, it will tend to slip. The inevitable consequence is poor decision making and unhelpful negotiating. When you report back to the board that you have achieved a good deal on transferring anticoagulant monitoring to general practice, only to be told that the GPs do not want to do it, that is the time to bite hard on your NHS dentures. Boards can be unforgiving creatures!

Mars and Venus

And do not assume that general practice has moved on further than it has in reality. The rhetoric of cross-partnership working, sharing resources and openness of information slips smoothly off the tongue but the Mars of competitive business may still be in ascendancy over the Venus of co-operating practices. We are faced with a continuing dilemma that is likely to take time to resolve. It encompasses independent contractor status and the clamour for equity. It balks at the concept of levelling down, at disincentives to innovation, at being identical to any neighbour and at losing income. It may be in need of a PMS pilot.

Personal medical services (PMS) pilots

PMS pilots, previously known as PCAPs (Primary Care Act pilots), are becoming more popular as they have become more attractive. This chapter is not long enough to deal with PMS in detail but will endeavour to outline the concept in broad-brush strokes.

The NHS Act 1977 has two parts, I and II. Part I deals with trusts which have local contracts with their host HA agreed annually. Part II deals with GPs and their pay under GMS regulations (the Red Book). The Red Book determines the fees and allowances payable to GPs and is hugely bureaucratic. But, and this is a major 'plus', under Part II of the Act, it is largely non-cash limited. In other words, however much GPs claim, they will be paid, provided that the claim is made in accordance with the regulations. (In fact, there is a national cash limit but this does not affect GPs' claims. It is regulated year on year by adjustments made through the Doctors and Dentists Review Body.) The cash-limited elements are staffing, cost rent, computing and primary care development. Prescribing budgets are also cash limited.

PMS allows practices to opt out of Part II of the NHS Act and be governed by Part I. The Red Book with its nationally negotiated rates is replaced by an annual local contract with the HA, entering the cash-limited Part I. This stipulates the quality standards that must be met under the terms of the contract. Whilst some of these are laid down nationally (e.g. vaccination and cervical smear targets), most may be locally set according the needs of the local community and the priorities of the local practice. Practices may choose whether or not the prescribing budget is added to the contract.

PMS Plus allows practices to provide some community services and some other HCHS-funded services as part of the contract negotiated with the HA. These too will be subject to quality monitoring on a regular basis.

Advantages

There are significant advantages for practices going the PMS route:

- reduction in the bureaucracy of claiming fees and allowances according to the Red Book
- the replacement of fees and allowances (with their arbitrary targets and activity-based items of service payments) by agreed clinical quality standards
- the clinical standards are flexible to suit local needs and can be varied year by year
- greater flexibility in practice arrangements, e.g. the ability to employ assistants rather than take on further partners without the loss of elements of fees and allowances
- with PMS Plus further appropriate services may be pulled into primary care using the HCHS budget.

Fears

There are fears acknowledged by some GPs:

- it is potentially uncomfortable to have your pay directly related to the profit remaining after medical care has been provided. For some reason many see this as different from the situation that pertains in normal general practice
- there are concerns that a hard-pressed HCHS budget will begin to suck money out of the primary care pot of money. This does not seem to have been a problem in any of the pilots to date and those involved say that the primary care pot is protected
- many dislike the fact that Part I of the NHS Act is effectively cash-limited and do not like to feel that they are moving out of a non-cash limited environment. As shown above, cash limits do operate and with time are likely to extend to more of GMS. A throwaway line in the NHS Plan refers to non-cash limited funds coming under the umbrella of a single resource allocation pot. How a non-cash limited pot can be

accommodated within a cash-limited pot without cash limiting it has yet to be ascertained.

Larger PMS pilots

Many practices have become PMS pilots on their own but it is becoming increasingly common for practices to join forces to form a larger pilot. This gains economies of scale, better risk management and greater negotiating power in setting the contract. Some areas have taken the concept further and formed PCG-wide (or nearly so) PMS pilots. This configuration is felt to give practices further protection against some perceived risks of PCT status. In some cases the PCT manages the PMS contract and in others it remains held by the HA.

One or two areas have gone even further and created large overarching partnerships covering a number of practices in a single PMS pilot. In at least one case this has served to keep practices in the same PCT when they are in a geographically distinct patch.

There is no doubt that a PMS pilot that encompasses a whole PCT provides a significant boost to integration across practices. Setting up the pilot and negotiating the terms of the contract takes the constituent partnerships through a process that greatly aids a mutual sense of ownership and co-operation. The advantages already outlined become even more secure with a larger pilot, though there must be a certain size at which the feeling of mutual ownership begins to be lost. It will be interesting to observe the progress of the larger PMS pilots to see how they fare.

CHAPTER 5

Clinical governance in primary care

David Lyon

When primary care clinicians first encountered the term 'clinical governance' in *The New NHS: modern, dependable*,[1] it was tempting to dismiss it as yet another soundbite, an oxymoron to file with 'virtually spotless', 'fresh frozen', 'military intelligence', 'friendly fire' or even 'New Labour'. What on earth, we asked ourselves, has the word 'clinical', associated with freedom, acumen, breakthrough and quality, got to do with 'governance', linked in our minds with command and control, regulation, administration and following orders?

However, in the consultative document *A First Class Service*,[2] clinical governance is at the core of the government's drive to improve the quality of the health service.

> *Clinical governance can be defined as a framework through which NHS organisations are accountable for continuously improving the quality of (their) services and safeguarding high standards of care by creating an environment in which excellence in clinical care will flourish.*

Many clinicians are sceptical about the impact on the reality of working with patients of a term whose definition sounds like a panacea for all the NHS's ills and includes the word 'framework'. However, *A First Class Service* provides us with absolute clarity when it states, 'For patients, the words "clinical governance" will mean better quality of care and greater confidence in NHS services'. This is the crux of the matter; patients will notice a difference.

Professional self-regulation, voluntary quality initiatives, such as clinical audit and the effectiveness agenda, and educational programmes, including professional development and mentor schemes, are recognised as valuable and important activities for clinicians. A lot of good, high-quality work has been done, with impressive results, and the government recognises this.

As it says in its supportive guidance,[3] 'The use of information, clinical audit, clinical effectiveness and continuing education are very familiar. Grouping the principles in this way, as part of a concerted programme of clinical governance within primary care, is new.'

Sadly, there are too many examples of bad practice, including outright clinical disasters, the closing of professional ranks to protect colleagues and inconsistent, unfair implementation of sound clinical evidence. Too few of us took part in quality improvement programmes with sufficient enthusiasm to make enough of an impact across the NHS as a whole.

It is our duty, individually and collectively, to demonstrate the quality of the services we provide. Clinical governance is the means by which we will do it. We should be excited at the prospect of being able to prove how good a job we do but there are those who do not like the sound of it. One thing is certain: if we don't make the best of it, there is something more draconian just around the corner.

Evidence-based practice

The art of Medicine is to amuse the patient whilst Nature cures the disease.

Voltaire

Voltaire was born 300 years ago and he obviously thought very deeply about the evidence base for medical practice. There have been fantastic scientific advances since then. There are scopes that can look into every orifice of the body and there are some that can create new orifices to look into. Surgical techniques include the use of lasers, diathermy, microscopes and fibre-optics. There are magic drugs for conditions as different as schizophrenia and peptic ulcers. There are even drugs for conditions which were not previously thought to have been diseases, such as obesity, the menopause and impotence. Nevertheless, Voltaire's observation is half-true. Nature still cures the disease but these days, the clinicians amuse themselves with their new toys.

In 1991, Professor Eddy wrote a famous editorial in the *BMJ*[4] which claimed that only 15% of medical activity was proven to work. A robust defence of the profession by our most eminent people managed to put this figure up to 30%. This means that 70% of what we do is unproven or known to do harm, yet we still do it.

Good clinicians, who care about what happens to their patients, should ensure they do the 30% that works, avoid doing harm and question the rest. First, the evidence base has to be searched to determine which activities work and which don't. Unfortunately, clinicians are bombarded with information, some of it accurate and some not, the majority from magazines and fliers or from visits by their friendly neighbourhood drug reps. They have little time to read the original papers themselves and few have critical appraisal skills even if they did.

Postgraduate education employs the use of a financial carrot to encourage GPs to continue their learning. Unfortunately, traditional medical education has failed to change clinical practice.[5-7]

The National Institute for Clinical Excellence (NICE) is designed to solve this problem along with the publication of National Service Frameworks (NSFs). Guidelines will be produced that review the research literature and make recommendations of those parts that should be implemented.

Only a few years ago, if someone went into a room full of clinicians with a ready-made set of guidelines, they would be chewed up and spat into all four corners of the room. The clinicians would then start afresh with a clean piece of paper and invariably come up with guidelines that looked remarkably similar to the original set. Everyone needed to go through the process of drawing up guidelines themselves in order to achieve ownership. These days, we are more mature and are happier scrutinising the work of others, making only a few adjustments to suit local requirements.

The process is likely to be slow. NICE has only just begun to organise itself. We are promised 30 new sets of guidelines a year. To date, very few documents have been published. The problems faced include the strength of the research evidence, the lack of which leads to the drawing up of consensus guidelines. If the consensus is decided only by 'experts' then the guidelines will bear little relation to the reality of working in primary care and will be harder to implement.

Implementing clinical change

Stocking[8] best describes the elements that influence clinical change. For change to occur, the general climate of opinion in the local, national or international environment has to be supportive. The change itself has to have perceived advantages for both professionals and patients by fitting in with existing beliefs and practices, by low complexity and by the ability of clinicians or patients to actually observe a difference at local level. The process in individuals and practices will vary, moving along a continuum from innovators, early adopters, early majority and late majority to laggards. The importance of immediate peers and colleagues is greater for the early majority than for the laggards. Local 'champions' are key change figures.

A multifaceted approach is an effective strategy.[9] Promoting Action on

Clinical Effectiveness (PACE),[10] Framework for Appropriate Care Throughout Sheffield (FACTS)[11] and the North West Regional Cardiovascular Disease Development (CARDD)[12] projects all came to similar conclusions:

- practices need support
- organisational change is necessary to change individual clinical behaviour
- a bottom-up approach that involves all those working at 'street level' is required
- practices are unique and will come to their own solutions but will learn from others
- a facilitator or 'change agent' is needed to drive the process
- resource issues, such as prescribing costs, clinician time and IT, have to be addressed
- barriers to change have to be identified and dealt with
- IT training is required, even in the most computer-literate practices.

In relation to secondary prevention of chronic disease, Schofield[13] identifies the structures needed as: protocols; disease registers; repeat prescribing systems; recall; structured records, such as computer templates; nurse-run clinics and training; patient education methods and materials; rehabilitation programmes and audit.

The biggest challenge for NHS managers charged with delivering clinical governance and PCGs or PCTs is the top-down, bottom-up conundrum. They have been given instructions on what to do by the government but clinical governance will only happen if those working in primary care believe in the process and 'own' it.

In the NHS there is a surfeit of 'transactional' managers who are top-down in attitude and who plan, budget and exercise control. They are often more concerned with process than outcome and are bureaucratic and mechanistic.

There is a shortage of 'transformational' leadership. This is characterised by charisma, inspiration, intellectual stimulation and individual consideration. 'Transformational' managers establish direction, motivate and lead by example. They develop teamwork, devolve responsibility and allow people to perform their tasks in the way they feel best. They appreciate the importance of relationships and take care to cultivate and nurture them.

It should be a compliment, therefore, that the management of the system is being devolved to PCG/Ts, closer to the clinicians and the patients. Here, we are looking for transformation or evolution rather than revolution.

Monitoring

The recent case in Bristol has illustrated the need for mandatory systems of identifying and correcting poor performance.[14] The GMC,[15] UKCC codes of professional conduct for nurses, health visitors and midwives,[16] terms of service for general practitioners[17] and the requirements of summative assessment[18] are no longer enough.

Evidence confirming satisfactory performance needs to be gathered and transmitted via practices' clinical governance leads to the PCG/T, the health authority, the regional authority and then to the Commission for Health Improvement (CHI), who will oversee the whole process. Patients and health professionals will be better informed and in a position to improve matters.

This may sound threatening for the average health professional. However, the system will have rules around both patients' and clinicians' confidentiality. The idea is to identify areas for improvement rather than to apportion blame. Individuals are accountable for their own performance but teams, practices and PCGs are accountable not only for their own performance but for its improvement.

Clinical audit should receive a new lease of life under these circumstances. There are high levels of participation by practices in clinical audit but not enough of it is linked to good evidence or to continuing professional development.[19] To date, clinical audit has been regarded as a voluntary activity outside normal core functions and the results are rarely acted upon. In the context of clinical governance, it is easy to imagine how an audit's results can form the basis of a PCG/T-wide discussion on the causes of any differences between clinicians or practices. The targets for the next cycle of the audit could then form the basis for corrective action.

In fundholding, the decisions were almost entirely the responsibility of the GPs. Now, nurses, health visitors, social workers and lay people are more involved. This is an ideal opportunity for real multidisciplinary, interagency work to enhance communication, support teamwork and enable joint decision making.

Complaints procedures in primary care have been changed so that more complaints are dealt with at practice level. There is a reporting mechanism to the health authority but it only examines complaints on a superficial level. Patients can also take their complaint to professional bodies or even to lawyers. It will take a great deal of trust for clinicians to share their experience of complaints, let alone near misses, with their peers in the PCG/T. However, we need to trust our peers to tackle the problem of performance monitoring adequately. The alternative is to leave it to outside scrutinisers.

CHI is meant to assist us to monitor and improve performance, with reference to the NICE guidelines and National Performance Frameworks (NPFs). We need not get too excited, as their initial budget is only going to be £4 million, compared to £100 million for OFSTED, and they're likely to be busy with acute trusts at first.

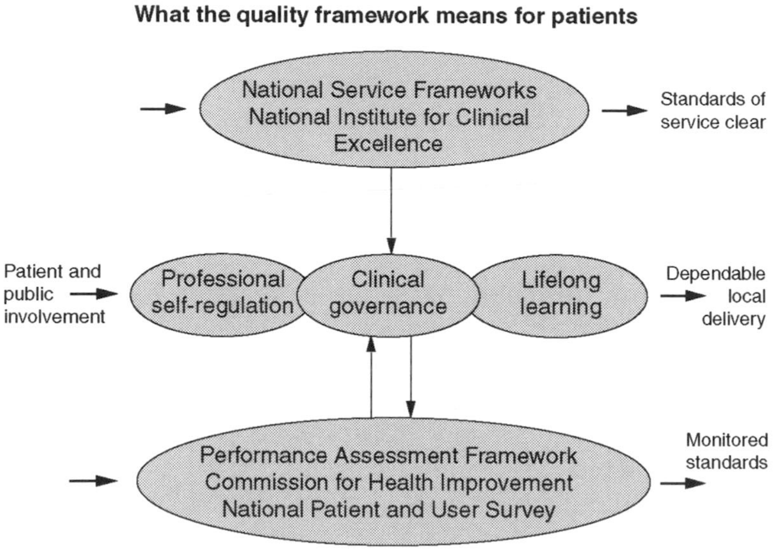

What the quality framework means for patients

Figure 5.1 Clinical governance framework.

Figure 5.1, from *A First Class Service*, illustrates clinical governance beautifully. It sits right at the centre. It is fed by the NICE and NSFs which will spell out clear standards of service. It is dovetailed with professional self-regulation and lifelong learning, with input from the public, so that local services can be seen to be dependable. Finally, it is supported by the CHI, NPFs and patient surveys, which will help monitor standards.

There are very particular tasks that need to be carried out by PCG/Ts that are detailed in *Clinical Governance: quality in the new NHS*.[20] The guidance is so crystalline, with specific deadlines, that the document needs to be read in detail by everyone involved in clinical governance.

The vision for the next five years for clinical governance to be successful involves health organisations, including PCG/Ts, being able to demonstrate:

- an open and participative culture in which education, research and the sharing of good practice are valued and expected
- a commitment to quality that is shared by staff and managers and supported by clearly identified local resources, both human and financial

- a tradition of active working with patients, users, carers and the public
- an ethos of multidisciplinary team working at all levels within the organisation
- regular board-level discussion of all major quality issues for the organisation and strong leadership from the top
- good use of information to plan and to assess progress.

There are four key steps.

1 Establish leadership, accountability and working arrangements.
2 Carry out a baseline assessment of capacity and capability.
3 Formulate and agree a development plan in the light of this assessment.
4 Clarify reporting arrangements for clinical governance within board and annual reports.

Leadership and accountability

By April 1999, the chief executive should have identified a clinician to lead clinical governance. This person was expected to assemble a team, probably with representatives from each practice, to develop different aspects of the programme.

Everyone should be involved and fully informed, there should be free access to the top, particularly to help overcome problems, and strong, open relationships with health trusts and other agencies have to be formed. There should be constancy of purpose, an ability to provide a comprehensive overview of progress and, most importantly, regular communication with everyone including external partners.

Baseline assessment

A fully participative PCG/T-wide assessment had to be made by the end of September 1999. As a minimum, it should have included:

- a searching and honest analysis of the PCG/T's strengths and weaknesses in relation to current performance on quality
- the identification of any problematic services
- an assessment of the extent to which data are in place for quality surveillance
- establishing whether there are deficits in key mechanisms (e.g. risk management, clinical audit, IT, patient participation)

- making sure that there is integration of quality activities and systems
- establishing links to HImPs, NSFs and locally identified priorities
- designing ways in which underpinning strategies (i.e. IT, human resources, continuing professional development) will support clinical governance.

Development plan

After the baseline assessment has been completed a plan has to be put in place. It should address gaps in the current performance, the development of an infrastructure (i.e. IT, human resources, continuing professional development, linkages with other organisations) and identify the training or development needs of the primary care clinicians and the PCG/T board and staff.

The plan should link closely to local HImPs and should be designed to implement NSFs.

Reporting arrangements

A reporting process has to be agreed with the health authority and a first annual report on clinical governance had to be published in 2000.

Three broad questions need to be answered.

1 Where did we start? (the baseline position)
2 What progress have we made and how do we know? (the development plan for the year and the monitoring and evaluation undertaken)
3 Where are we going next? (the development plan for the coming year).

The reality of the coalface

The task is frighteningly huge and the deadlines painfully short. How can PCG/Ts, and particularly the clinical governance leads, possibly deliver all this in reality? There are no streams of funding or manpower flowing from a hitherto undiscovered spring.

However, we need to bear in mind that the overall vision is laudable and something all reasonably minded practitioners would want to aspire to anyway. If we don't do it, then someone else will come along and do it for us. No-one is better placed than ourselves to understand and assess primary care. We can carry out the baseline assessment and develop and implement an action plan much more sensitively using a more 'transformational' approach.

There is already a lot of high-quality work being done. The idea is to bring together all quality activities so that 'the whole is greater than the sum of the parts'. Most practices participate in clinical audit, many have worked out ways of engaging patients in the process, the Royal Colleges have energetic programmes devolved to local level and postgraduate education is well organised and often has close links to hospital and community trusts. The nurses, health visitors, midwives and other professionals have well-developed activities of their own.

Some PCG/Ts have devised standard questionnaires for practices to complete and others have held meetings for representatives from each practice but the best results are achieved if they are all visited for a face-to-face discussion. This is an opportunity for the whole team to have their say about how they see things going and how they think things can be improved.

General practices are the building blocks of PCG/Ts and are the bases where most of the clinical work will be carried out. Practices are long-standing organisations and often have a very clear idea of their goals and objectives. They also house a wealth of information for a baseline assessment. It is ideal if the practices feel that their views are valued and acted upon.

Clinical governance action plan

PCG/Ts will already have developed an action plan. Hopefully, the practices' views will feature prominently in it.

Many of the action points will be allocated to existing subgroups within the PCG/T structure. Others will have to be dealt with by the clinical governance team.

An action plan might look like this.

Multidisciplinary team working

Although many practices have a tradition of multidisciplinary meetings, it may be necessary to re-energise them and encourage a change in culture in other practices. The clinical governance will have to find training for the practice leads to enable them to co-ordinate, build teams and ensure good communications within the practice and with the PCG/T. All the practices could use a rotating agenda including: practice professional development plans (PPDPs), clinical topics derived from the HImP, clinical audit results, peer review and video consultations, risk assessment and critical case analysis.

Clinical audit

This should be multidisciplinary and multipractice and the cycle needs to be completed. A systematic approach needs to be applied to the whole PCG/T. The topics should come from the HImP, preferably led by those involved in the HImP subgroups and supported by the multidisciplinary audit advisory group (MAAG). It would be fruitful to plan one or two interface audits with the trusts engaging with their audit staff.

Evidence-based practice

Often there will be locally agreed guidelines in place and there will be other areas with a demand for one. Clinical topics are the easiest way to get clinicians from different organisations talking to each other. There may be a desire for a journal club and the practices need to have a mechanism to scrutinise those national guidelines thought to be important or most relevant to general practice.

Prescribing

There will be a subgroup looking at prescribing anyway. There will be an aspiration to agree a formulary and to introduce safe and robust repeat prescribing mechanisms. Clinical audits could be driven by a prescribing need.

Risk management

The clinical governance team may need to improve communications between clinicians from different organisations, as this is the most common reason for dissatisfaction on both sides. There may be a primary care development subgroup, which could lead on risk assessment and critical event analysis. The Medical Defence Union risk management pack is an excellent resource.

IM&T

There is bound to be a subgroup for this as it is the only area for which there are resources available. Practices will need training on Read coding (the most common computer code for recording clinical information in primary care), will need help recording significant events that occur away from the practice and may want computer templates to help collect data systematically in nurse-led chronic disease clinics. This is quite apart from the equipment and a skilled person to obtain and analyse data from all the different systems. Arrangements have to be made to fulfil the national requirement for Caldicott guardians.

Commissioning

The visits to the practices will have produced a list of services which need improvement in terms of access or quality. These ought to be passed on to the commissioning subgroup for action.

Patient and user involvement

This is an issue for the PCG/T as a whole. It is likely that the lay member of the board will be chairing a group to address how to engage with the public meaningfully. Practices need to support the process, perhaps by inviting some of their patients to make a contribution.

Training and development

It makes sense to pull together all the different training organisations to develop a co-ordinated approach across the PCG/T. This will include PPDPs for all grades of staff in primary care, team building, clinical audit training, nurse training in chronic disease management, peer review and mentoring, critical appraisal, receptionist development, tutorials or case studies, postgraduate qualifications and the provision of 'protected time'.

This list may seem daunting, but if the plan has been drawn up by consulting with practices and other agencies in an inclusive, bottom-up manner, then it is realistic to expect progress in all areas. Many of the action points can be added to the agendas of subgroups. This is perfectly reasonable as clinical governance should drive every aspect of the PCG/T's activities. It would be wise to have at least one member of the clinical governance team on each subgroup to ensure that the clinical governance plan is implemented.

A progress report should be delivered to the board in six months with regular updates in between. An annual report has to document progress and revise the plan accordingly.

The example of ischaemic heart disease

Ischaemic heart disease is one of the four government priorities and is one of the topics for the HImP. It is covered by a comprehensive NSF.[21] The part that is most relevant to primary care is tabulated on page 11.

People with cardiovascular disease should:

- *have those risk factors which can be reduced assessed and documented*
- *receive information about their risk factors and the scope for reducing these*
- *receive advice about how to stop smoking including advice on the use of nicotine replacement therapy*
- *receive appropriate medication, on the basis of the available evidence, including:*
  - *low-dose aspirin for those with proven atherosclerosis*
  - *beta blockers for those who have had a heart attack in the past year*
  - *ACE inhibitors for those with left ventricular dysfunction*
- *have their blood pressure maintained below 140/90 mmHg*
- *have their blood cholesterol concentrations lowered to less than 5 mmol/l and LDL-C below 3 mmol/l or by 30%.*

The final document is a very clear summary of the available evidence, so that clinicians will not have to look any further to verify what should be done.

The NSF will work best if it is implemented in the 'transformational' manner, using a bottom-up approach as described above and illustrated in CARDD.

Each practice should be visited in order to establish how cardiovascular disease is dealt with at present. Most will have a clear idea as to what should be done clinically, some will have arrangements in place for people to have checks by a practice nurse, some will record data on the computer and others will have criteria for referral to secondary care. Few will have a systematic approach, although, on discussion, the vast majority will agree that it is a good idea.

The next step is to invite interested parties to a general meeting to discuss cardiovascular disease. It is important to ensure that all groups are represented, especially practice nurses, managers, IT people and doctors. This group could then be facilitated to deliver the NSF.

The likely outcome is an agreement to have a disease register for call and recall to a nurse-led clinic where the relevant interventions can be carried out and recorded on a computer template or easily auditable paper template. Any identified as having difficulties would be referred to the GP, who could adjust medication, organise further tests at an open access clinic or refer for secondary care assessment, according to an agreed local guideline.

The disease register could be drawn up for the repeat prescribing records, which are generally computerised. Those on nitrates are a good first group to search. Their paper record needs to be put onto the computer to ensure they are called and recalled. This already identifies a need for practices: someone with a basic IT knowledge to computerise the notes and create the register. The knowledge required is different for each computer system. The health authority's primary care information strategy group should have access to the human resources required. Sometimes, the local multidisciplinary clinical audit group will have expertise in this area. Once the register is set up, an administrator needs to be identified to keep it up to date and to invite patients for review.

A nurse resource needs to be identified to review the patients. This could be shared between practices or could be drawn from nurses carrying out tasks of lower priority, for example well man clinics. The health authority could again be a source of help but the local community trust may be more useful, as blending district nurse and practice nurse roles could release nurse time.

These nurses need training in the management of heart disease and the use of the computer systems. Nurses, GPs and secondary care doctors should get together to decide the protocol for the nurses in the clinic and what happens outside it. The hospital doctors need to know how to get patients back into the primary care system and the role of cardiac rehabilitation needs clarification.

The GPs need to be clear about prescribing and the PCG/T needs to be aware that the biggest cost is going to be the statin drugs.

Professional education on heart disease could be offered to all members of the primary care team across the whole PCG/T via the local consortia or even with the support of drug companies.

The vast majority of computer systems have a template facility to ensure the systematic collection of data. IT training and help is a problem for even the most computer-literate practices. Many MAAGs have developed computer templates for cardiovascular disease and many IT computers provide training on how to use them. Certainly, the audit of those in the disease register needs to be thought about at an advanced stage, with a set plan including deadlines. Targets could be set for patients reviewed, proportion on aspirin, cholesterol levels and even number of myocardial infarctions or hospital admissions, etc.

The availability of open access exercise tests or echocardiograms is an issue for referral protocols and commissioning. Often a standard referral form could be used and the service could actually be run by a GP or nurse practitioner with a special interest who is willing to be trained and employed as a clinical assistant. This service, although ostensibly a secondary care one, could be audited along with the practices.

Smoking clinics can be agreed upon and run PCG/T-wide, focusing on those areas of greatest need. Negotiations with local leisure facilities and health promotion units can lead to exercise-on-prescription programmes. Healthy eating programmes can be put in place and the problem of the availability of cheap, healthy food in deprived estates can be addressed with local authorities. People with chronic disability can be identified and fed into the Benefits Agency and citizen advice in order to ensure they receive all the benefits they're entitled to. The physical shock of a heart attack on a middle-aged man is bad enough, but the loss of a breadwinner has disastrous effects on the whole family.

A focus group of patients with heart disease and their carers can inform the whole process and a survey could help monitor the service.

As each practice will be at different stages and have different requirements to implement the NSF, resources have to be directed towards need in order to achieve equity. This does *not* mean everyone being given exactly the same resources. Once the disease registers are in place and are reasonably accurate, the need for drugs, tests, nurses and hospital attendance can be determined fairly. In addition, it will help with establishing the need for services from other agencies.

Thus, with the example of heart disease, we can see how the whole process of clinical governance works.

Clinical guidelines are issued from the NICE or a NSF

↓

The service is reviewed locally beginning at practice level

↓

Relationships between all interested parties are developed

↓

A system is set up to ensure all the relevant interventions are delivered to all the relevant people

↓

Resource problems are addressed

↓

Commissioning is better informed

↓

Professional education and training are focused according to need

↓

Patients are actively involved in the process

↓

Other agencies, including secondary care, community trusts, health authorities, the voluntary sector, the local council and the multidisciplinary clinical audit groups, are actively enlisted to help

↓

Audit is carried out to demonstrate benefit

Advantages of being a primary care trust

A PCT's access to a real budget will make it easier to implement the action plan. Resources could be identified to support the multidisciplinary meetings at practices and to support the clinical governance links' development needs.

Many of the action points will only be enacted if the subgroups are effective. In PCGs, these groups are almost dependent on the goodwill of the participants whereas a PCT could resource them appropriately. 'Protected time' is an important issue for clinicians whose time and skills are best suited to seeing patients. This issue is not being properly addressed by PCGs but could be by a PCT.

Many of the solutions will involve additional clinical time at practice level. In the example of IHD, the nurse time was a crucial element and this is likely to be the case for many chronic diseases including diabetes, hypertension, respiratory disease, epilepsy, rheumatoid arthritis and heart failure.

Imaginative solutions to waiting list problems could more easily be carried out by a PCT. For example, a couple of GPs could be trained in orthopaedics and provide a primary care clinic to assess patients from all practices. They could establish a relationship with the surgeons so that they could list patients directly or order NMR scans, etc. These GPs would be able to engage with practice-based physiotherapists and provide a management plan for their own doctor to follow as appropriate. This approach has the potential to reduce the demand on outpatients and free the surgeon to spend more time doing joint replacements. Such a suggestion might be taken up by a co-operative health authority after due consultation but a PCT has power over its own destiny.

Drug companies

PCGs might have to resort to begging from drug companies. Most of the research evidence that is clear proves the effectiveness of medication. A key aspect of clinical governance is to implement the research evidence in a systematic manner. For most diseases, this will mean an increase in prescribing both in numbers and in cost. If the chronic diseases are being optimally treated 30% of the time, practices will be doing well. When clinical governance works, drug companies will make bigger profits because there are very few areas where there will be reduced prescribing.

It is a good idea to ask groups of companies to sponsor projects. Those that produce statins could be asked to pay for extra heart nurse time. The guidelines will drawn up without their help but will be implemented more quickly. The PCG will have to be open and accountable about its relationship with companies.

In addition, drug companies would be wise to provide support to clinical governance generally, not just to clinical areas for which they make products. Supporting multidisciplinary meetings and developing the clinical governance practice links will benefit them as well.

As part of the deal, the clinical governance lead could ask the companies not to send drug reps to practices. The idea is to move away from the clandestine, mysterious encounters that take place in surgeries or restaurants or, even, the Orient Express. A relationship that can be more easily scrutinised and will benefit patients more easily is far better.

Conclusion

Clinical governance is an exciting new initiative by the government. It will enable clinicians to drive service changes in order to improve the outcome for patients.

The vision for the future is clear and the steps for the implementation of clinical governance are explicitly set out. It is seen to be at the core of the NHS, so quibbling over it being 'non-core' in respect of general practitioners' terms of service is spurious.

It will be supported by the National Institute for Clinical Excellence, National Service Frameworks, the Commission for Health Improvement, National Performance Frameworks and National Patient and User Surveys. However, most importantly, the whole of the NHS will be dovetailed to interact with it.

The process of clinical governance will bring together quality programmes, such as audit, professional education and regulation in a more co-ordinated manner to involve all clinicians constructively. In addition, the NHS will be better able to work with outside agencies to improve health.

All clinicians, especially those in primary care, should welcome this opportunity to make a difference for their patients. It is time we rolled up our sleeves and got on with the work before someone else decides to do it for us.

References

1 Department of Health (1997) *The New NHS: modern, dependable*. The Stationery Office, London.
2 Secretary of State for Health (1998). *A First Class Service*. Department of Health, London.
3 Department of Health (1998) *The New NHS: modern, dependable: primary care groups: delivering the agenda*. Department of Health, Leeds.
4 Eddy DM (1991) What care is 'essential'? What services are 'basic'? *JAMA*. **265**(6): 782, 786–8.
5 Sackett D, Rosenburg W (1995) On the need for evidence-based medicine. *Health Economics*. **4**: 249–54.
6 Davis D, Thomson M, Oxman A and Haynes R (1995) A systematic review of the effect of continuing medical education strategies. *JAMA*. **274**: 700–705
7 Oxman D, Thomson M, Davis D and Haynes B (1995) No magic bullets: a systematic review of 102 trials of interventions to improve professional practice. *Can Med Assoc J*. **153**(10): 1423–31.
8 Stocking B (1992) Promoting change in clinical care. *Quality Health Care*. **304**: 56–60.
9 Bero L, Grilli R, Grimshaw J *et al*. (1998) On behalf of the Cochrane Effective Practice and Organisation of Care Review Group. *BMJ*. **317**: 465–8.
10 Dunning M, Abu-Aad G, Gilbert D, Gillam S and Livett H (1998) *Turning Evidence into Everyday Practice*. King's Fund, London.

11 Eve R, Golton I, Hodgkin P, Munro J and Musson G (1997) *Learning from FACTS. Lessons from the Framework for Appropriate Care Throughout Sheffield (FACTS) project*. ScHARR, Sheffield University, Occasional Paper 97/3.

12 Elkind A, Lyon D (1998) Practice makes perfect: changing clinical behaviour in primary care. *Br J Health Care Manage*. 4(10): 484–8.

13 Schofield T (1996) *Secondary Prevention of Heart Disease in Practice*. Primary Care Heart Save Project, Oxford.

14 Smith R (1998) All changed, utterly changed. *BMJ*. **316**: 1917–18.

15 General Medical Council (1998) *Good Medical Practice*. General Medical Council, London.

16 United Kingdom Central Council for Nursing, Midwifery and Health Visiting (1992) *Code of conduct for the Nurse, Midwife and Health Visitor*. UKCC, London.

17 Department of Health (1992) *National Health Service (General Medical Services) Regulations 1992. Schedule 2. Terms of Service for Doctors*. HMSO, London.

18 Conference of Postgraduate Advisers in General Practice (1996) *Summative Assessment: general practice training*. National Office for Summative Assessment, Winchester.

19 Hearnshaw H, Baker R and Cooper A (1998) A survey of audit activity in general practice. *Br J Gen Prac*. 48: 979–81.

20 Department of Health (1999) *Clinical Governance: quality in the new NHS*. Department of Health, London.

21 Department of Health (2000) *National Service Framework for Coronary Heart Disease*. The Stationery Office, London.

CHAPTER 6

Delivering community services to the benefit of patients

Robert Sloane

Perhaps the only test of the government's modernising reform programme should be of the tangible benefits that are brought to us all, as citizens, members of families and communities and of course as taxpayers.

The tendency to become preoccupied with the new organisational frameworks – primary care groups and primary care trusts – as if they matter is quite understandable. But keen enthusiasts of primary and community care development will see them for what they really are – a transitional means to an end rather than an end in themselves.

The end which this chapter anticipates is one which concerns itself much more with the holistic well-being of individuals and communities in order that they remain in a state of independence for as long as possible.

A new philosophy

To contemplate the potential of the new community-orientated changes requires a major shift in traditional NHS thinking.

- Only the citizen as part of the wider community can effectively constrain his or her demand for increasing levels of care. Responsibility for health and social well-being must primarily be a personal one. It is the duty of government and its agencies to facilitate the maintenance of health and then to ensure that adequate and appropriate provision is made when individual and collective effort is not sufficient.
- It is this fundamental shift in responsibility from government and its organisations to the citizen and their communities which is inherent in the idea of maintaining health as opposed to curing illness.

- The pivot of the new community orientation is the home, supporting people in varying degrees of wellness and when necessary organising care in and around where they live. On the one hand maintaining independence and a sense of personal responsibility for as long as possible, on the other, utilising the global community resource which is the very fabric of which society is composed.
- Although the definition of community varies, people in general feel some sense of where they belong: a street, a parish, a town or just an entity which has a label attached to it. Although more difficult to spot in the large urban areas, a basic sense of community is often more evident than a superficial examination might suggest.
- With the new definition of health and wellness must come a recognition that health systems do not and cannot exist in isolation. The success of the community service model will depend on the degree of horizontal integration with other statutory and voluntary agencies.
- Increasingly, in the new environment the skills of all staff will remain key. A new equation will be drawn with a closer connection between health needs, which will determine what form of competence-based response is mobilised. Many existing staff never utilise their capability to the full and are often constrained by unchallenged professional dogma about how services should be organised.

Quite clearly, from what has been said, the focus of care is expected to move even closer to where people live and work, i.e. home and community (Figure 6.1). The trend has been in this direction since the early 1990s, but much of the NHS has yet to catch up. Differences between the 'new' and 'old' order might be expressed in the following way:

'New' order	'Old' order
home	hospital
community	institution
health promotion	curative service
needs led	supply side driven
team competence	professional individualism
participation	prescription
multiagency	unisystem
independence	dependence

Even now it is easy to forget that 93% of contact with the health service takes place in primary care.

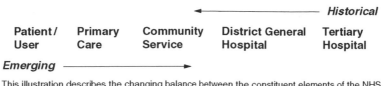

This illustration describes the changing balance between the constituent elements of the NHS.
It also depicts the continuum of care which begins and ends in the patient's own home.

Figure 6.1   The changing context of the NHS.

PCTs in context

It is this 'new' order which has set the strategic backcloth for the development of PCGS and PCTs. The creation of PCGs was the first phase of the government's plans to modernise the NHS in conjunction with modernising policies affecting all aspects of public service. At the local level there has been an explicit expectation that health services would work in a more 'joined-up' fashion with Social Services, education, housing and other statutory agencies.

Specifically, PCGs recognise that family doctors and community nurses are usually the first port of call for patients who need advice or treatment and they are also responsible for referring patients into the rest of the NHS.

PCG functions

The stated overall functions of PCGs chime very much with the 'new order' outlook:

- improving the health of the community
- developing primary and community health service
- commissioning secondary care services.

An Audit Commission briefing of February 2000 illustrated how a number of PCGs had gone about their business to good effect by:

- contributing local evidence to health planning
- gathering data to plan primary care investment
- co-ordinating services
- employing pharmacists to help GPs make more efficient use of drugs
- setting up programmes of interpractice audit and learning
- agreeing targets and making board decisions in public.

Satisfying as these innovations are, it is the prospect of further patient-centred change which has led many PCGs to embark on the progression towards becoming PCTs.

PCT functions

Official guidance specifies:

> *Primary Care Trusts (PCTs) will be new, free-standing, statutory bodies with new flexibilities and freedoms, responsible for delivering better health and better care to their local population.*
>
> *They will have their own budget for local healthcare, be able to employ staff and develop new integrated services for patients. They will undertake many of the functions presently exercised by Health Authorities, for example commissioning health services, investing in primary and community care and improving the health of the local population.*
>
> *PCT status brings added freedoms and opportunities to develop integrated services that are responsive to patient needs.*

According to the Audit Commission report, the most common, positive reason given by aspirant PCGs for seeking trust status was the opportunity for further local service integration and greater flexibility in community care development. Some viewed a trust application as the natural consequence of having a strong community spirit, proactive GPs and a desire to develop community hospitals. Others saw benefits in direct funding. There could be better opportunities to develop primary care, with speedier implementation of plans and fuller control over the local health economy.

Rationale for movement to PCT status

Those contemplating the move towards trust status will need to be clear about the freedoms and attendant responsibilities within the new accountability framework.

At a headline level the areas where PCTs might be expected to make a difference could include the following.

Health improvement

- Developing locally responsive services, giving patients better access to healthcare by identifying where services most need developing. This will be achieved by taking the health needs of the community as the start point for planning and commissioning of services.

- Improving local rehabilitation and intermediate care services, reducing the need for patients and relatives to travel to an acute hospital.
- Fostering interagency partnerships to establish new forms of community governance.
- Constructing locally owned services that recognise and build on the contribution of voluntary organisations, utilising community networks.

Development of primary care

- Agreeing investment and disinvestment priorities for practices.
- Developing professional development and career opportunities on a multidisciplinary basis.
- In line with the Local Information Strategy, meeting the information needs of practices by supporting investment in appropriate practice-based information systems.
- Supporting GPs in clinical audit, research and teaching.
- Offering alternative employment models for GPs who wish to take them up.

Public participation

- Strengthening locality links with the Community Health Council to give local people the opportunity to influence the shape of local health services and contribute to the decision-making process.
- Being proactive in the assessment of local views on healthcare issues.
- Adopting an open style of business conduct in relations, which stimulates interest and involvement.

Quality and clinical governance

- Delivering a clinical governance agenda will assure high-quality services and create the opportunity to build on existing clinical governance structures in community services and the PCG.
- Promoting a culture of lifelong learning through continuing professional development.
- Supporting GPs in clinical audit, research and teaching.

Value for money

- Developing federated support services to practices:
  - IT support
  - payroll services
  - HR advice
  - education, training and development
  - HR services such as agency and bank.
- Sharing infrastructure costs with Social Services and local authorities.
- Providing joined-up service solutions utilising budget flexibility.
- Maximising the use of limited resources and minimising the impact on patient care of potential disinvestment.

Arguably, one of the most tantalising attractions of the PCT mechanism is the potential to completely redefine the model of safe and cost-effective local services.

The evidence base of the HImP and the locus of the weighted capitation budget will together create a powerful new dynamic which is both of the community and in the community.

A close analogy might be of an electromagnet when the current is turned on. The resultant field force will help to energise horizontal integration between local partner organisations and attract services into a community setting.

Many would argue that the commissioning clout of a PCT level 3 organisation would be sufficient by itself to bring about change of this nature. The contention of this chapter, however, is that only the synergy of integrated commissioning and providing can assure the full potential of the local service model.

In this functional fusion lies the essence of the new incentive structure of a unified health and social care system. At the base level, thinking will be more about 'providing in primary care what you can and commissioning what you can't'.

Testing the community services model

How the new set of levers impacts on the community services model will differ from one location to another and be governed by a range of factors. Not least of these will be:

- the historical basis of collaborative working
- the broad acceptance and readiness for change
- shared ownership and responsibilities between stakeholders

- extent of a shared vision
- acceptance of the need for managed change
- current patterns of morbidity.

Any suggestion that there might be a shortcut to an 'idealised' form of community service 'blueprint' (or that this chapter might offer one!) is to be resisted at all costs.

The starting point will be different in every instance. History, current evidence, vision, partnership working and the occasional mistake are essential in the cultural proving, which cannot be hastened.

However, it might be helpful at this stage to contemplate a process which could help to inform the logical basis of any community services model. This involves the application of a test matrix to determine the most appropriate placing of services in the future. Although Table 6.1 refers to a typical range of existing community services, the test matrix can equally be applied to new and evolving services.

Table 6.1 The community services 'menu'

Category	Services
General community nursing	District nursing Health visiting School nursing Family planning Midwifery
Community PAM services	Chiropody/podiatry Dietetics Speech and language Sexual health Community physiotherapy Community occupational therapy Rehabilitation services Audiology

Specialist community services	Community dental
	Specialist nursing: stoma care
	Palliative care
	Diabetes
	Continence
	Specialist clinical:
	    geriatrics
	    paediatrics
	    gynaecology

Table 6.1 The community services 'menu' (*continued*)

Category	Services
	community psychiatric nurses/teams
	Drug/alcohol Services
	Dermatology
	Rheumatology
'Facility' based services	Community hospitals
	Intermediate care:
	hospital at home
	prevention of admissions⎫
	early discharges ⎬ working with SSD
	Vulnerable people/long-term care beds
	Day hospitals
	Minor injuries
Other	NHS Direct
	Social care
	Transport
	Management of waiting lists
	Out-of-hours primary care
	Wheelchair services
	Equipment loans services
Functions	Human resources
	Finance
	Information technology support
	Training and development
	Corporate functions

The test matrix

Before to the commencement of testing it will be essential to assess the current scope and capacity of local primary care and particularly to understand the threshold between primary and community care. This will inevitably be a complex interface involving a range of factors: clinical, financial, managerial and socioeconomic. Of particular importance will be a mapping of the referral pathways which lead out from primary care (Figure 6.2).

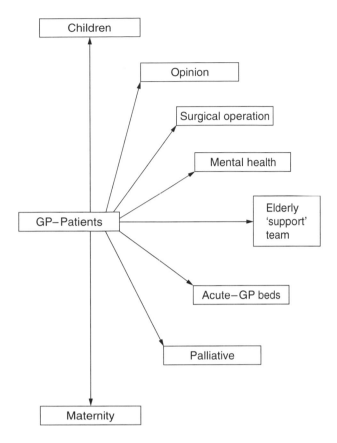

Figure 6.2   Referral pathways.

Initial audit

For each of the existing services it will be necessary to begin with:

- the name of the service
- the staff by grade and number
- the catchment area
- extent of relationship with primary care
- key service linkages external to the trust.

This will be a preliminary to a fix on the key linkages within the trust, the range of skills and competence involved in providing the service, the means of clinical supervision and the basis of continuing professional development.

This initial charting stage will in many cases already have been under-taken in the form of a service prospectus or similar documentation.

Assessment criteria

With the initial audit completed a series of criteria need to be applied to decide the configuration of component services.

- *Evidence of need.* Is there a demonstrated need for the service evidenced by the HImP or a substantiated justification of commencement/continuation?
- *Stakeholder support.* Are partner organisations prepared to fund/continue funding the service in the present/proposed configuration?
- *Fitness for purpose.* Are the services provided in relation to need or dimensions of geographical, socioeconomic, demographic and care groups?
- *Integration.* Is the service integrated with those from other relevant agencies and professionals? Are scarce resources and skills maximised?
- *Safety.* Can high-quality clinical services be provided that will meet the standards set locally and nationally by professional bodies, National Service Frameworks, etc.?
- *Cost effectiveness.* Does the service offer value for money, economies of scale?
- *Auditability.* Can the care pathway be tracked and all the elements involved in the service assessed?
- *Staff fitness.* Do the staff have appropriate levels of competence, experience and training? Do all staff have clinical supervision?
- *Employer status.* Is there demonstrable employer capacity, i.e. human resource capability? Do staff have access to and support for continuing professional development?

Community hospitals

Perhaps a particular reference could be made at this point to the role and function of community hospitals. A strong argument is advanced for their reclassification as community resource centres and therefore prequalified candidates for inclusion in the community services model.

In the majority of instances community hospitals have evolved from a strong sense of community and are regarded as touchstones of the local NHS. They have multifaceted integrating roles which include:

- health-promoting activities including leisure and lifestyle
- first point of local access for ambulatory care
- combining GP out-of-hours and minor injuries service now augmented with NHS Direct

• easing pressure on acute services through active rehabilitation programmes.

Increasingly, these roles will expand, assisted by the advent of new technologies including near-patient diagnostic testing and telemedicine.

Organisational framework

Only when the service model (i.e. function) is determined should attention turn to form, i.e. the most appropriate organisational framework. In this latter respect the range of options for consideration might include:

• incorporation within the PCT
• hosted from one PCT and provided to others
• provided from a single healthcare organisation.

Although this is a provisional list there may be scope for hybrid agency arrangements to develop.

Conclusion

To recap on an earlier theme, the wide variation in starting points means that there will not be one single model for the organisation of community health services and the effect of the development of PCTs will be multifaceted. Given the potency of the integrated commissioning/providing model, it seems highly likely that the PCT level 4 will gain ground in short order.

Many of the PCT's functions are currently being undertaken by community trusts. The immediate challenge for health authorities, trusts and Social Services is to continue to provide integrated, efficient community service throughout a time when responsibility for these services is being transferred from established organisations to emerging ones.

With the PCT comes enormous scope to do things differently, in accordance with the third way. Although definitions vary, the 'third way' is a sort of hybrid middle course between the fragmenting contestability of the internal market on the one hand and the stifling effects of centralist planning on the other.

In essence the 'third way' is about finding new ways of creating whole-system change based on perceptions of mutual benefit.

The new PCT incentive structure provides for a more integrated approach to be taken at the local level. The legitimate focus on primary and community care excellence should, in theory, allow other parts of the health system to concentrate solely on those functions for which they are uniquely equipped.

Producing joined-up solutions, particularly where this involves local pooling of resources, including budgets, results in better outcomes for clients/patients at lower cost.

The real test will be the extent to which resources can be moved within the whole-system approach. This is likely to be problematic. But on it will rest the scope to achieve new models of care and retain the professional interest of those developing them.

CHAPTER 7

Commissioning and providing for PCTs

Roger O'Brien Hill

Introduction

The commissioning of care services is much more a matter of evolution than revolution. There are good reasons why change in either the way that we commission care or where we commission care from must be approached with a great deal of caution. The number of influences on the way we commission services grows from year to year. Broadly, the issues that will influence the way in which PCTs approach the commissioning process can be grouped thus:

- impact on hospital infrastructure
- clinical accreditation/governance
- finance
- being both a purchaser and provider of secondary care services
- the primary/secondary care interface
- the effect on other commissioners
- National Service Frameworks (NSFs)
- central government priorities
- NHS/Social Services integration
- prescribing as part of the unified budget (i.e. can reduce available HCHS funding)
- national and regionally set targets
- Health Improvement Programme (HImP).

The pros and cons relating to these matters will be discussed in more detail throughout this chapter. PCTs will pick up the mantle of being the host commissioners from the health authorities and partnership with the local trusts will be key to successful commissioning.

In the past, health authorities have seen their main priority as balancing the books and have therefore concentrated on closing the financial gaps with trusts rather than the volumes of specific services that are commissioned. In addition, the protection of their host trusts has been paramount. Fundholders, however, concentrated on buying specific services in the volumes they required, with less regard for the trust from which they purchased the service. The price and quality of individual procedures were the major deciding factors, not the financial impact on the trust. In future, PCTs will have to balance the priority of obtaining value for money with that of maintaining the financial stability of their host trust. In addition, PCTs will be expected to invest in, and develop, primary care.

Commissioning acute services

The changing nature of acute services offers an opportunity for PCTs to redistribute funding. Over time, funding may be released for investment in primary care in a variety of ways. These include: higher day-case rates, shorter lengths of inpatient stay and improved surgical techniques such as better quality prostheses, minimal access surgery, improved drug regimes, the transfer of some hospital-based outpatient services to the community and better GP control of initial referrals.

In the short term most PCTs will have inherited a very tight financial regime from their health authority, with an increasing range of national and regional targets to be met (e.g. waiting lists, outpatient waiting times, CABG and other NSF targets) that will not only reduce local flexibility but will have to be achieved within the available financial envelope. Here are some ways in which these often conflicting priorities can be balanced.

- Work with your trust to benchmark their services against other trusts and use the information to seek improvement where performance is below the national benchmark. The National Benchmarking Club might be able to help.
- Use the National Cost Reference Database to determine how your host trust compares with others on a financial basis. This data is available on a CD-ROM held by your health authority.
- Seek to develop outreach services in a community setting rather than allowing your trust to expand their infrastructure. Remember that most of a trust's cost lies in staff, buildings and equipment, not in the amount of activity that they deliver on behalf of any individual PCG/T.
- Remember that referrals = activity so if you can meet the expectations

of the patient in other ways (e.g. GP-to-GP referral, prescription, etc.) then you will reduce demand on the secondary sector.

- Use long-term service agreements (LTSAs) to give you and the trust the opportunity to plan services better and with less financial risk.
- Review the low-tech hospital services such as dermatology, minor surgery, endoscopy, etc. to see if there are alternative outreach settings from which services could be provided (e.g. larger primary care centres).
- Seek to review the way in which diagnostic services are provided to reduce repetition and delay.
- Work with other agencies such as Social Services to co-ordinate services in the community to assist in reducing the need for medical beds and achieve the discharge of patients from those beds at an earlier date.

In general, PCTs wishing to shift major volumes of activity from one trust to another will have to accept that this activity can only be removed at marginal cost. In any circumstances the best opportunity to effect large-scale change will be when a trust is seeking to make a step change in its service provision. Proposed new buildings, increases in staff and the proposed purchase of new equipment always offer the opportunity to review the way those services are provided before committing to the new spend/growth and may offer the opportunity to remove cost at full value.

Relocation of patient activity from outlying hospitals can also reduce your costs. This can be achieved by:

- a reduction of out-of-area treatments (OATs). The cost savings will be delayed for two years due to the way that OATs funding works. Be wary of increasing your OATs activity; although in the short term it could save money it will reduce both funding and flexibility in the longer term
- a reduction in the number of service level agreements (SLAs) that are placed with trusts. This will avoid being locked into fixed-cost SLAs where activity is volatile
- the use of a 'traffic light' type system including a single page summary as an *aide-memoire* to inform and assist your GPs when making referrals and to ensure that they are directed to the provider where the appropriate SLA has been placed (i.e. green = main provider, orange = alternative cautionary provider, and red = specialist provider).

In the longer term, when waiting lists are no longer the focus of national attention, prioritisation of patients on a needs basis rather than length of wait will provide a better and more equitable way of determining the length of wait for elective procedures. Patients will only be placed on a waiting list when their need has been established and once they are on a waiting list, their procedure will be carried out in a much shorter length of time.

Attention needs to be given to the number of outpatient appointments attributable to an individual referral (first to follow-up ratio). These can be influenced in the following ways:

* not referring to secondary care in the first place (e.g. by GP-to-GP referral)
* referring for an opinion only
* follow-up appointments being done by GPs
* shortening waiting lists (long waits for procedures often result in more outpatient appointments)
* encouraging consultants to return patients to the care of their GP.

Commissioning specialist and tertiary services

Although GPs do not normally refer direct to tertiary services they will, through the placing of SLAs, have the opportunity to direct these referrals to a provider of their choice. In many cases it may just be a matter of consolidating the activity for your PCT and directing it towards one provider but it could also lead to some financial benefit.

In the current PCG environment, PCGs will have chosen to levy back funding and commissioning responsibility for most specialist services to their health authority. However, in the future as health authorities merge and become more distant and PCTs gain more commissioning experience, much of this responsibility will fall to PCTs. The key issues relating to the commissioning of specialist services are:

* risk (financial volatility from year to year)
* cost of individual episodes of care
* ensuring that a satisfactory provision is maintained and financed
* economies of scale (i.e. consortium approach with other PCTs).

Commissioning and providing community services

The commissioning of community services is where the big opportunities for rationalisation will lie as PCGs move to PCT status. PCTs will take responsibility for the management and provision of all community services and as a consequence, community trusts will disappear with their mental health responsibilities being merged into larger mental health trusts. There will be scope to redefine the delivery of these services around new community hospitals or primary care centres to offer a better, more integrated, near-site set of services.

There will be opportunities to review the delivery of nursing, including the integration of district nursing and practice nursing services. This will be further enhanced by the introduction of nurse prescribing and nurse practitioner status. Nursing teams offering a more seamless, consistent and integrated service are likely to be the most cost-effective way of delivering the services in the future. Factors likely to drive nursing integration are:

- clinical governance
- shortage of nurses
- shortage and cost of GPs
- finance.

Specialist nursing will often be provided by a few highly skilled nurses where it is unlikely that one PCT could provide a financially viable service and sharing with other PCG/Ts would be sensible. It would also be sensible to operate a 'knock-for-knock' type of agreement where treatment of patients from other PCTs is necessary. School nurses are an example, providing a service to all the schools in an area regardless of the PCT to which the children 'belong'. Attempting to cross-charge each other for these services would create an administrative nightmare.

Services provided by professions allied to medicine (PAMs) are already available in both community and practice-based settings. The provision within practices largely arose as a result of fundholders who often favoured in-house services. However, this has often given rise to inequities between former fundholders and non-fundholders. There have been increasing pressures to move towards equitable levels of service provision without either increasing or reducing the level of services provided. This could be achieved by providing near-site services made available to the patients of all practices and by allocating usage targets to each GP/practice. This in turn will lead to equity between practices within a given service provision and also give GPs visibility of their usage of the individual services. This solution could equally apply to psychology and counselling services although it remains unclear who would control these services – PCTs or mental health trusts.

Services for older people could be more of a problem for PCTs to manage. First, if the services are taken on by the PCT, there are issues around the capabilities of PCTs owning and managing beds which will massively increase both their complexity and infrastructure. However, if a PCT chooses to take all other community services except services for the elderly, who will manage these services? Community trusts will disappear as all the other services are taken on by PCTs and mental health services will remain entirely separate.

Services for older people should be provided as near to the community as possible, which does favour the PCT taking ownership along with the strong Social Services link. The management of beds for the elderly could also be the key to controlling the number of acute beds occupied by the elderly. These beds, along with GP beds in the management of the PCT, could also operate as a 'step-down' bed facility for acute patients following major inpatient procedures.

Practice-based services

Practice-based services will already exist in all PCTs but may have historically been provided without any wider planning. Former fundholders usually purchased services to meet the needs of their practice populations. This presents PCTs with several problems.

First, whilst most GPs have seen in-house services as offering better, more accessible care to their own patients, it is difficult to provide an equitable service to all patients in a PCT in this way. Generally, an expansion of the service throughout the PCT would create significant cost pressures.

Second, some of these in-house services will be provided by a random selection of private providers with sometimes inadequate professional supervision, ongoing training and cover. At worst, some practitioners may be found to be insufficiently qualified to provide the service in the first place.

Third, some of the services can be described as alternative medicine. Careful consideration must be given as to whether these services should be provided at a cost to the NHS. Many alternative therapies have their detractors and may not be acceptable to all professionals who may feel other priorities are more pressing. Extending such services across a PCT may therefore be fraught with difficulty.

Finally, funding sources will have varied, from GMS funding, fundholder savings, management funding to non-recurring funding and finally HCHS funding, all of which will now need to be rationalised.

Thought needs to be given to how these services can be provided in a more equitable, cost-effective and acceptable fashion. The term 'near-site' might offer a solution. Providing these services on a shared basis, with access to all, at a site near to each practice (e.g. community centre, local hospital or one GP practice) could offer a number advantages:

- equity for all patients
- proximity to patients
- cost efficiency
- more economic use of clinicians' time (i.e. less travel)
- reduction in the use of private providers
- reduction in the need for special equipment at multiple sites.

Commissioning services for people with learning disabilities

People with learning disabilities (PLD) are usually a small, well-defined group and their needs are usually provided for by a well-defined service. Patients with learning disabilities are often identified early in life and often in hospital or by a health visitor. However, it is a shared service with much of the resource being provided by Social Services, but a significant number will have associated clinical conditions requiring medical intervention such as mental illness, cardiac conditions and physical disabilities.

Although the number of patients registered as learning disabled is relatively small, their needs are lifelong. In the last decade improved care has resulted in the average life expectancy of learning-disabled patients increasing dramatically, with a consequential rise in the cost of supporting these patients. However, costs can be contained by identifying the appropriate care packages throughout the patient's life.

In the first place it is important that a shared register of all PLD patients is maintained. It will be necessary for the information on all PLD patients to be understood at practice, PCT, trust and Social Services level. It will be important to ensure that patients moving in and out of the PCT area are tracked.

Learning-disabled patients can be broadly grouped into four categories:

- those requiring support to maintain their quality of life but with no real expectancy of any improvement
- those who, with the right package of care, can be expected to show an improvement in the quality of their life
- those who currently do not require any support (e.g. children supported by their parents) other than that due to an ordinary NHS

patient but who can be expected to require learning disability services at some time in their lives

- those who are classed as volatile, who would not normally need care but who may require short periods of intensive care

The key to managing commissioning for PLD is the patient. All patients should have expectations clearly defined, as above, and have an individual, clear care package with outcome expectations identified, along with a named lead care worker for each patient. It will then be possible to price the packages of care and monitor outcome against expectations.

Commissioning mental health services

Mental health services are unlikely to come under the control of PCTs in the foreseeable future and may well be provided by a larger out-of-area mental health trust. The NSF for mental health will ensure that the services retain a high level of visibility and consequentially carry a high level of risk. This will increase the difficulties of providing a locally focused and integrated service with Social Services.

Co-terminosity of CMHTs with local Social Services and the PCT to provide a locally focused community mental health service will be essential. Arrangements will need to be made with the mental health trust to ensure that the CMHTs can be properly managed with a local focus and are seen as a local service and not part of the owning trust. CMHTs will act as a gatekeeper to the more expensive acute mental health services.

Management of mentally ill patients in the community is handled by the care plan approach (CPA), which places patients into one of three categories. Each patient has a care plan and a named lead worker and the management of patient movement on and off a CPA as well as movement between CPAs is an excellent way for all parties to monitor their patients. In the same way as for PLD patients, a shared list of patients on a CPA should be maintained at practice level.

Some mental health services (e.g. forensic) will need to be provided on a PCG/T-wide basis to reduce risk for any individual organisation, due to their cost and volatility.

Information requirements for commissioning

Information is essential in managing any process but even more so when managing the process of providing a cost-effective, balanced health service to a defined group of patients.

The most important information is provided via the contract minimum data set (CMDS). This record should define every single patient interface with commissioned services (i.e. outpatient, procedure, diagnostic test, PAMs appointment, etc.). For each individual piece of activity, it will define who attends, where they came from, what was done to them and how much it has cost. If this information is complete (which it is not at the moment) then all the other necessary analysis to conduct the commissioning and monitoring processes can be derived from it.

Data will be used to determine the size of your unified budget and distance from target. These in turn will produce the HCHS financial envelopes that will be the basis from which you will start all commissioning. Important data analysis requirements are shown in Table 7.1.

Table 7.1 Data analysis requirements

Data type	Data type detail	Source	Use
Practice list sizes	Age/sex breakdown	Exeter system	PCT list size and management budgets
	ASTRO PUs	Derived	Prescribing allocations
	York formula weighting	Derived	HCHS allocation/DFT
CMDS	Diagnostic	Acute trust	Commissioning/monitoring
	Outpatient	Acute trust	Commissioning/monitoring
	Inpatient	NWCS*	Commissioning/monitoring
	Community	Community trust	Commissioning/monitoring
Practice	Activity	CMDS	Practice comparison
	Prescribing	PPA	Performance
Bed days	Acute	Acute trust/NWCS*	Commissioning
	Mental health/PLD	Mental health trust	Commissioning
	Elderly/GP	Community trust	Commissioning
A&E		Acute trust	Sizing

*NHS-wide clearing system

Service level agreements and performance monitoring

Service level agreements will need to not only reflect the normal activity assumptions but also meet the requirements of the national and regional targets that have been set. Remember, any trust will prefer to have only one set of quality and performance parameters to work within, so it would be sensible to encourage PCG/Ts to agree on a single financial envelope and a joint SLA with their host trust. The larger the financial envelope within your SLA, the less the financial risk to individual PCTs.

Activity data provided by trusts has on the whole been provided late and has been poor quality. Now is the opportunity to build into the SLA both the data requirements and the timing of receipt of the information. It might be possible to tie in a financial incentive for the trust for providing accurate and timely data. The guidance for 2000–1 makes it clear that the trusts have a duty to provide accurate data to PCTs at both a PCT level and a practice level.

Conclusion

In summary, the key points to remember when you are commissioning services are as follows:

- GPs are the gatekeepers to almost all commissioned services
- getting your correct share of the budget is vital
- accurate timely information is a valuable tool
- limit your risk by sharing with others
- you must achieve the nationally set targets
- watch the timetable.

CHAPTER 8

Public health and PCTs

Siân Griffiths

Introduction

Primary healthcare has traditionally been focused on the care of individual patients whilst public health has been concerned with the health of populations. Not so long ago their futures could have been characterised as developing in parallel with very few crosslinkages. However, with the current programme of modernising the NHS one of the key changes has been to give primary care responsibility not only for healthcare but also for the health of the population. The new structures proposed, whether PCGs, PCTs or some other configuration, will all have public health responsibilities. They all have responsibilities for improving health, developing primary care and commissioning services to promote the health of their population.

This chapter will explore some of the implications for the mutual development of primary care and public health. It will consider the historical roots of public health, how they intertwine with primary care and the challenges the new agenda sets for their future development.

Historical roots of public health

Public health is best characterised as a population perspective on the health of local communities. Other key aspects are:

- an emphasis on collective responsibility for health and on prevention
- recognition of the key role of the state, linked to a concern for the underlying socioeconomic determinants of health as well as disease
- a multidisciplinary basis which incorporates quantitative as well as qualitative methods
- an emphasis on partnerships with the population served.[1]

The definition coined by Sir Donald Acheson: 'The science and art of preventing disease, prolonging life and promoting health through the organised efforts of society'[2] highlights that, contrary to some common perceptions, public health is not just about health promotion through prevention but also about the organisation of services to promote effective and efficient models of healthcare delivery.

Origins of public health

The current structure of public health has emerged from historical roots in the 19th century. Tracing the role of one of its lead actors, the director of public health, helps us to understand some of the complexity of the current role.[3]

The first medical officer of health, the redoubtable William Henry Duncan, was employed in the city of Liverpool just over 150 years ago. For the rest of the century the preoccupation of MOsH who followed him was environmental improvement and sanitary reform; campaigning for improved housing conditions, the supply of clean water and better working conditions, particularly of industrial workers. Key to their work was the collection of statistics about their populations, particularly about births, deaths and disease. As government legislation began to promote the public's health through a series of Acts of Parliament, the focus of public health widened from environmental concerns to include personal health and social care: mother and child health, immunisations, care of those with chronic infectious diseases, care of the mentally ill.

To quote from the recent history of the NHS by Rivett:

> By 1968 MOsH had a smoothly running empire, managing community nursing service, social work services, the aftercare of people who were mentally ill or handicapped, the ambulances and the child and school health services.[4]

However, in 1974 the role of medical officer of health was changed. Leaving local government, MOsH joined the NHS as district community physicians (DCPs). Public health nurses who worked in community health services also moved into the NHS, leaving behind other public health practitioners including environmental health officers and social workers. As community physicians, PH doctors increasingly became part of NHS management. With successive reforms DCPs became district medical officers (DMOs) with a focus on hospitals and medical management. However, their nadir came in 1989 when the government introduced the purchaser/provider split and for many, public health became synonymous with the antagonistic contract negotiations between hospitals and health authorities. Following the Acheson review in 1997, they were renamed directors of public health in recognition of the need to regain their wider role in promoting the health of communities.

During this time others with public health roles were developing in diverse and unco-ordinated pathways. Community nursing and the relationship with general practice underwent significant changes, not least the introduction of practice nurses and of practice attachments for health visitors and other community nurses. These new arrangements reflected the shift away from the local government mother and baby clinics and family visiting to greater responsibilities within primary care for some of the key tasks of public health such as immunisations and screening. General practice began to play a major role in public health through the new arrangements for health promotion, for which GPs received target-related payments.

Yet the relationship between public health physicians and general practice has often been strained, with PHPs being accused of focusing on the acute rather than the community sector and primary care practitioners being accused of looking after their practices, not their local populations.

Criticisms of public health were not the sole territory of primary care. The chief medical officer had recognised in 1988 that there was:

- confusion about the role of public health doctors
- concern about the organisation of control of communicable disease
- a lack of emphasis on health promotion and prevention
- a paucity of population-based information on which to base policy decisions about the health of the population
- poor capacity in health authorities to look at outcomes and priorities.[2]

His report suggested solutions which were encouraged by the change in government in 1997, since when public health in the UK has had something of a renaissance.

Public health at the beginning of the new millennium

The day after the election of the Labour government in 1997, a new post, that of Minister of Public Health, was created. This symbolic appointment signalled the concern not only for health services but also for the factors which impact on the health of communities: environment, education, poverty, housing. The relationship between these factors, the same ones that were the concern of the early public health pioneers, and health was once more open for debate.

Setting the scene: two important policy initiatives

Amongst her first actions, the Minister for Public Health commissioned the *Independent Inquiry into Inequalities in Health* chaired by Sir Donald Acheson.[5] She also launched the process to produce the White Paper *Saving Lives: our healthier nation*.[6] Both documents are relevant to the inter-relationship between public health and primary care trusts.

The Acheson report

The Acheson report[5], an *Independent Inquiry into Inequalities in Health*, was commissioned to review the latest available information on inequalities and health and to identify areas for future policy development. Although the primary focus of the report was to make policy recommendations to the government on a wide range of issues, including the structure of tax systems, housing, ethnicity and transport/mobility, it also addressed the structure of the NHS. There were two key aspects of primary care which received particular comment: equity of access and resource allocation.

Equity
The report highlighted the finding that communities at risk of ill health tend to experience the least satisfactory access to the full range of preventive services, in line with the inverse care law. Prevention services include cancer screening programmes, health promotion and immunisation. Differences are most noticeable among socioeconomic groups but other factors also impact on equity, for example ethnic group. It is likely that additional inequalities in access are experienced among Bangladeshi women. To quote the report:

> Lack of access to women practitioners can deter Asian women taking up an invitation for cervical cancer screening. Local studies show that access to women practitioners is poorest in areas with high concentrations of Asian residents, and practices are less likely to reach their targets.[6]

Resource problems

The resource problems of inner-city areas are well known. It is more difficult to recruit doctors into deprived areas and poor premises make this
worse. In London, health promotion claims are highest in least deprived
areas. Thus the report recommends action to redress these inequalities
with needs-based weighting to GMS resources.

Saving Lives: our healthier nation

Saving Lives is the government public health strategy published in the
summer of 1998 following extensive consultation. In its foreword the
Prime Minister states:

> *I believe that by working together we can tackle poor health and achieve
> the aim of better health for everyone, and especially for the least fortu-
> nate ... The White Paper is a significant step towards better health. It
> sets out a new modern approach to public health – an approach which
> refuses to accept that there is no role for anything other than individ-
> ual improvement, or that only Government can do something.*[6]

The White Paper, which sets out the strategy for public health for the next
10 years, is summarised in Box 8.1.

Box 8.1   Summary of *Saving Lives: our healthier nation*

AIM is to improve the health of everyone and the health of the
worst-off in particular.

KEY MESSAGES
• **Tackling inequalities**
  Poverty and social exclusion recognised as major contributors
  not only to poor health but also to inequalities in health and
  society. Root causes need to be addressed not just by the NHS
  but by action in all sectors and at all levels.

• **Emphasis on role of government for social, economic and
  environmental factors**
  National and local need for joint working to address determinants of ill health formally recognised by a duty of partnership.
  Introduction of health impact assessment for all policies.

- **Balance of action for people, communities and government**
  Emphasis now is on the interaction between individuals, communities and government working together.

- **Targets**
  National
  Four key areas at national level for the major causes of death: cancer, CHD, accidents and suicide. Variety of other strategies: alcohol, HIV/AIDS, tobacco, teenage pregnancy, communicable disease.

  Local
  To be set by HImPs.

- **Emphasis on the important role the NHS has to play: evidence-based effective practice**
  Environmental and socioeconomic issues are important but effective healthcare also makes a contribution to improved health. Issues about effectiveness, access, appropriateness and quality of care are important in improving quality of life.

- **Developing the capacity of the NHS and others to deliver this agenda**
  - Strengthen public health nursing.
  - Recognise the contribution of multidisciplinary public health, developing training and accreditation to allow career progression to consultants/DsPH.
  - Invest in PH academics.
  - Strengthen PH research.
  - Ensure better co-ordination of the PH network.
  - Develop an education and development strategy.

Implications of the public health agenda for primary care

Tackling inequalities in health

Understanding the health needs of a local population requires the collection and collation of information. The information may be quantitative, such as that provided by the public health common data set and routine data sources including health visitor records, or it may be qualitative, such as the information obtained from focus groups or questionnaires. Comparative analysis between affluent and poor areas will show poorer health status for the less well-off. Outcome of action to address this gap should be measured on a routine basis. PCTs will have a major responsibility in addressing local inequalities.

Emphasis on the role of government: national and local

In the past there have been assumptions that improvements in health can be achieved either by individuals taking responsibility for themselves or by governmental regulation. The emphasis within *Saving Lives* is on the integration of individual responsibility and governmental regulation with community responsiveness and action, giving rise to the well-known phrase 'joined-up government' at national level, which acknowledges that the cycle of deprivation will not be broken by actions of the health service alone. Concerted action to reduce inequalities by promoting opportunities for better education, more jobs and less poverty as well as more accessible health services is needed. Additional resources for health action zones (HAZs), healthy living centres and projects such as Surestart and Young Offender Trailblazers reflect central government commitment to this approach.

At a local level, joint working between health services and local government has been promoted by policy which encourages joint working. For example, *Partnership in Action* promotes the discovery of new and flexible ways of sharing resources, such as pooled budgets.[7] Local authorities have a responsibility to consider within their community plans the health impact of social, environmental and economic factors. Primary care organisations and local authorities are increasingly working together to respond to local need. Examples such as exercise on prescription, joint bids for lottery money, shared initiatives in local schools and greater involvement in housing issues reflect some of the moves that have been made. PCTs within HAZs can take an active role in neighbourhood renewal and social regeneration agendas and projects. Community nurses, particularly health visitors, have an important role to play in such initiatives.

Targets: national and local

Targets have been set at national and local level. The national targets are set to combat common killers. Public health departments monitor progress towards the targets as an integral part of the performance management process. All PCTs need to know what their contribution is to the overall targets. In addition, they may, within the HImP process, set themselves local targets. These may not be just about death as an outcome but may be about well-being or about process. Public health professionals will usually be involved in helping PCTs to establish and monitor these targets.

Evidence-based effective care within the NHS

Evidence-based effective practice is part of the quality agenda. Throughout *Saving Lives* runs the assumption that research will be put into practice. Constraints on doing this lie in awareness of the research findings, lack of systems for their implementation and the inevitability of prioritisation and rationing that this presents. Whilst PCTs are well placed to address local issues, advances in tertiary and specialist services may pose more of a problem. Public health practitioners have a key role to play in providing the evidence to help balance the various demands of prevention and care and secondary and specialist services. Public health skills underpin the implementation of National Service Frameworks and the development of critical networks.

Developing capacity

The emphasis on capacity building refers not only to public health departments and the need for multidisciplinary public health practitioners. Although PCTs will have an interest in the development of public health departments which meet their needs, they will also have direct concerns about developing the public health skills of their staff. Across the country there are a variety of initiatives to increase the public health skills of those who are public health specialists, such as health visitors. PCTs also have a developmental role in supporting those who have an interest in public health, such as GPs and members of PCT boards. Good use of available education resources can underpin a strategic approach to developing public health skills. Developing capacity also requires strong links with academic departments and the creation of effective networks for communication and shared learning.

What has public health to offer?

Against this scenario, how can existing public health resources best be used? The practice of public health is continually evolving and the modernisation agenda recognises the need for continuing and rapid evolution as the NHS becomes primary care led. At present PCG/Ts have access to public health skills from:

- their local public health department
- their own practitioners
- other public health practitioners, e.g. environmental health officers
- local academic departments/institutions
- national bodies.

Local public health departments

Each health authority has a department of public health which is headed by a director of public health who is a medically qualified executive director on the board of the health authority. Other staff in the department include the consultant in communicable disease, other medically qualified public health consultants, specialists in public health qualified in a variety of areas such as health promotion, information and health economics and others such as analysts and specialist nurses working in control of infection.

The core elements of a public health practice have been defined by the Faculty of Public Health Medicine.[8] Their application to a district is described below, with examples of relevance to PCG/Ts.

Surveillance and assessment of the health of the population
Includes:

- the DPH annual report
- health needs assessment
- monitoring change, particularly in reducing inequalities.

Example
The annual report of the director of public health is produced each year. This year the focus is on mental health. The report contains local maps that show which electoral wards in the district have higher numbers of homeless people. Research shows that homeless people have greater mental health problems and therefore need targeted services. The PCT has a high rate of homelessness and is taking the report into account as it

prepares its primary care action plan. It has also requested additional information from the public health department. Together with the local authority, the PCT has employed a project officer to assess the level of drug abuse among homeless young men and assess their needs. The project will use the model from a nearby district described as best practice in the report. The results will be included in the next annual report.

Protecting and promoting health and well-being, including communicable disease control and environmental health
Includes:

- specialist health promotion support
- communicating/listening to the public
- acting as an advocate for the public.

Example
The government has published its tobacco strategy and every practice in the PCT must have a smoking cessation lead person. The health promotion specialist with responsibility for reducing heart disease has worked with the chief executive of the PCT to identify and train the practice lead. She is also offering ongoing support about effective interventions and collating the statistics on cessation from the practices.

- Surveillance of outbreaks.
- Emergency planning.
- Strategies for control of infection.
- Monitoring immunisation uptake.
- Health input into environmental health issues.

Example
The consultant in communicable disease control (CCDC) leads the team who monitor infectious disease for the district. Last week there were two cases of meningitis in the district. The patients were reported by the hospital to the public health department. The CCDC contacted the GPs of the patients, young men who both worked at the same factory but lived within different PCT catchment areas. All PCTs in the district were asked to be vigilant for suspected cases amongst others in the workforce. The CCDC handled the press enquiries, sending copies of press releases to the PCT chief executives. She used the opportunity of press interest in meningitis to promote the school-based immunisation campaign.

Managing knowledge and getting research evidence into practice
Specifically:

- applying evidence and research findings to local health issues
- synthesising local information, national policy directives, e.g. NICE and clinical evidence
- contributing to IT and information strategies.

Example
One of the greatest challenges facing health practitioners is how to manage knowledge. Muir Gray[9] estimates there are as many as five innovations in knowledge and technology in a single bi-weekly journal. Given the large number of journals and the exponential rate of knowledge development, help is needed to ensure appropriate policies are developed. The local public health institute runs training in basic epidemiology, critical appraisal of evidence and access to evidence. The PCT has decided that all board members should attend these courses. In addition, a database of local guidelines has been made accessible to all surgeries by the PH information team.

Managing, analysing and interpreting information and statistics
Includes:

- analysis of health data by condition, population group and geographical area
- providing information to a wide variety of organisations including PCGs, local authorities and trusts.

Example
The assistant director of public health leads the health information team. She and her team have produced a report for the PCT of referrals for elective procedures by practice. The CE of the PCT is using this report to discuss significant variations across the trust. Other PCTs have heard about this and want their analyses. Fortunately, in producing the information, the team anticipated this demand and did not need to repeat the exercise a further four times. However, this has been used as an opportunity to create a steering group to agree priorities and share work between PCTs in the district.

The team has also worked with the local authority to produce a directory of data sources which can be accessed by practices in the PCT. Public health support in accessing and using this data is available.

Developing and influencing policy
Includes:

- ensuring that national strategies are put into practice, e.g. the coronary heart disease National Service Framework
- developing district-wide health impact statements with local authorities, PCTs and trusts.

Example
The deputy director of public health is leading the group who will ensure the implementation of national guidance on the prevention and treatment of heart disease across the district. The group has representatives from primary care – one of the chairs of a PCT, a nurse from another and a lay member. It also has a consultant cardiologist, a senior hospital manager, a non-executive of the health authority, a member of the CHC and a health promotion specialist from a local authority.

The group has reviewed the expected targets for the district and identified several areas of weakness. For example, in the inner-city area there are higher than expected emergency admissions for coronary artery bypass grafts, especially amongst social class V patients. The local PCT is asked to review access for patients from its least affluent areas and to alert the GPs of the possible bias in their referral patterns. The practice nurse will work with representatives of the local Asian community to ensure that they know about the symptoms of heart disease and that they should seek advice at an early stage from their GPs. Advocates will be available to attend clinic appointments and act as translators for those who are less confident because their spoken English is not very good.

At the same time, the 'door to needle' times for anticoagulation patients in the rural parts of the county are too long and the respective PCTs are working with the ambulance trust on strategies to reduce this. Public health are providing relevant information and monitoring improvements.

Professional advice
Includes:

- liaison with medical directors and other senior clinicians in primary and secondary care
- understanding the district-wide perspective on medical workforce issues.

Example
The PCT chairs meet on a regular basis with hospital trust medical

directors. The meetings are co-ordinated by the director of public health. The agenda is constructed around issues of professional concern about the interface between primary and secondary care. This month there is particular concern about coping with winter pressures. Concerns include discussion of the threshold for and appropriateness of referral for admission from the community. Simple suggestions to improve communication were taken on board by the trust medical director.

The new directive for cancer patients was also discussed at the meeting. Views were sought from the GPs about how the new hospital system to make sure all patients are seen in two weeks is working. The DPH ensures that key points from the discussion are widely disseminated and follow-up action identified.

Working with all sectors which impact on health and healthcare
Includes:

- strategic shaping of health services to meet population needs
- clinical and epidemiological input
- clinical input into commissioning including specialist commissioning.

Example
There is general concern about the referral rate for endoscopy for diagnosis of peptic ulcer. The specialist registrar in public health works with the GP lead and senior clinician from the trust to review the epidemiology of helicobacter disease and the evidence for the various tests and treatments. New guidelines for referral are agreed and implemented. The specialist registrar evaluates the change in practice which results from the intervention.

Strategic leadership for health across all sectors
Includes:

- working with local government, voluntary organisations, commerce, criminal justice system
- supporting and developing the HImP.

Example
The health authority is charged with co-ordinating the HImP for the district. The director of public health is the lead executive for the HImP. She has regular and ongoing contact with CEs and key contacts from the PCTs as well as those from trusts, local authorities, the community health council and voluntary agencies. Increasingly, the five PCTs in the district choose priorities and take actions with their local district councils which

respond to local needs. This produces variations across the district. With the information team, the DPH and other health authority colleagues balance the national 'must dos' as laid out in the national priorities guidance with the locally derived plans which are important to local people. As part of this, PCTs are asked to provide health impact statements. The methodology for HIAs has been developed by a multidisciplinary, multisectoral project group of the HImP board. In addition, the views of local communities about priorities are sought by the public involvement groups of the PCTs.

Prioritising in health and healthcare
Includes:

- within the HImP and within commissioning
- utilising clinical effectiveness, evidence-based approaches and critical appraisal
- assuring local values are taken into account as well as national directives.

Example
The local healthcare system has a common forum for discussing new treatments and agreeing rationing decisions within the local health authority patch. Each of the local trusts has a representative on the forum. A new drug for treating cancer has been receiving wide publicity. Patients are approaching their GPs for advice. The local cancer specialist attends the forum to explain the benefits derived from results of randomised controlled trials. He also presents the costs. The DPH chairs the meeting and draws the forum's attention to the evidence of effectiveness, to the relative cost compared with other treatments purchased and to the national guidance. A decision is made not to fund the drug. This decision is communicated via the public health team to all GPs within health authority boundaries on behalf of the PCTs. This enables GPs to draw on the health authority statement when having to tell patients a potential treatment is not available.

Developing quality and an evaluative culture
Includes:

- taking an overview of clinical governance
- implementing recommendations from NICE
- acting as appropriate in relation to poorly performing doctors (the role here will become clearer with the development of the CMO's proposals).

Example
A GP with an interest in quality of care has been seconded to the public health department. His role is to bridge the gap between the health authority, who take an overview of the healthcare provided, and local practice. He is working with the local postgraduate education committee, the primary care audit group and others to improve the local performance against targets for the NSFs for coronary heart disease and also asthma.

Education and research
Includes:

- within all settings – community, primary care, hospitals
- with all stages and all disciplines: undergraduate, postgraduate, CPD.

Example
Medical and nursing students often have projects which involve statistics on the local patch. The PH information team can make local statistics available electronically to support their needs. In addition , the consultant and specialist staff contribute to learning sets for PCT staff who are interested in developing an understanding of public health.

Public health resources within the PCT

Public health resources in PCTs come via arrangements with local public health directorates. These include sessional commitments, SLAs, secondments and identified sources of specialist advice.

With the emergence of PCTs, formal public health advice to the executive is required. In addition, there are existing resources within PCTs and community trusts. Community nurses are often trained in public health, particularly health visitors and school nurses. A recent publication from the national health-visiting body recognised that the health-visiting role is at a crossroads and needs to define itself in relation to prevention of health problems in populations, communities, families and individuals. This implies a change to a more leading and enabling role, towards primary prevention for communities and populations through working with children and families. Since PCTs have responsibility for improving the health of their populations and addressing social inequalities, they will increasingly rely on community nurses to undertake the role.

The expected competencies of the public health person on the executive board are that they should be able to provide strategic advice, have knowledge of factors affecting health and disease, understand needs assessment and use of information, be competent at appraising evidence, be able to assess quality and effectiveness of health services, be familiar with health promotion and community involvement approaches and understand healthcare services. In addition, the person is expected to lead the development of public health within the PCT and have access to PH support outside the PCT. They should be able to work across boundaries at a strategic level, supporting involvement of hospital clinicians and contributing to prioritisation and management. The implication of these competencies must be a close link with existing PH departments, although the nature of the relationship is unclear. Some PCTs may seek to establish their own PH teams, although it will not be possible to disestablish PH depts.

Some functions which should not be delegated include arrangements for public health surveillance (including the prevention and control of communicable disease), maintenance of cancer registries and most functions under the Mental Health Act. Other functions need full consultation.

Public health resources in local authorities

Local authorities have clear public health roles in relation to housing, environmental health, education, Social Services and other services such as leisure. In addition, some authorities have designated public health posts. Some would argue that local authorities could and should provide the centre for local public health with expertise and support. This can be a sterile argument. What is needed is close working between agencies responsible for the same population and greater clarity of the contribution – the health impact – made by local authority decisions, policies and actions to local health status.

Active engagement with PCTs via their boards is one way of bridging the gap. Another is by shared projects and secondments as well as joint participation in setting and monitoring local targets set in the HImP, where possible making them the same as those in the local community plan. Training for public health practitioners as well as educational events for those interested in public health, such as elected members, are one way of increasing understanding of local public health issues.

Public health resources in academic institutions

Most PCTs will have access to local academic public health support. Although this may be available from medical school departments of public health, many other universities will have academic staff and students with an interest in population health issues. Schools of geography have an interest in mapping inequalities, sociologists are interested in patient/public perceptions of health and economists in the cost effectiveness of different models of care.

National public health resources

As well as local sources of support, there will be a national system of support for developing effective public health practice. For example, the Health Development Agency, previously the Health Education Authority, will advise on setting standards for public health and health promotion practice. Their website will carry information about effective health-promoting practice. Public health observatories are being established in each region of England to collate and provide public health information to all local bodies. The Cochrane Collaboration is available online and access to data electronically is being promoted via the National Electronic Library for Health.

The future

It is clear that PCTs have a public health role and that the relationship between public health and primary care is changing rapidly. Local public health departments are already changing the way they work, for example by agreeing SLAs, identifying specialists to support individual PCTs, establishing PCT PH learning sets and creating joint posts. This is a time of opportunity, of finding new ways for all public health specialists to work together, but care must be taken that it is not interpreted as a time of threat, of disestablishment of public health. Public health practitioners from all sectors need to find ways of working together to develop their professional skills, particularly those necessary to help PCTs succeed in their key role of improving the health of the population. As PCTs develop, the whole of the healthcare system needs to consider the most effective and efficient way to ensure good public health practice. Innovative solutions and joint working will be essential to achieve this aim.

> There is an urgent need for strong leadership at local level to improve health and reduce health inequalities. Primary care teams can be expected to play an active role, but not to lead. This must come from health authorities, whose job it is to provide strategic direction, to promote local action to improve health and health care, to reduce

inequalities and to support PCGs and the emerging primary care trusts.[8]

References

1 Beaglehole R and Bonita R (1997) *Public Health at the Crossroads.* Cambridge University Press, Cambridge.
2 Acheson D (1988) *Public Health in England.* HMSO, London.
3 Griffiths S, and Hunter D (eds) (1999) *Perspectives in Public Health.* Radcliffe Medical Press, Oxford.
4 Rivett G (1988) *From Cradle to Grave: 50 years of the NHS.* King's Fund, London.
5 Department of Health (1998) *Independent Inquiry into Inequalities in Health.* Chair: Sir Donald Acheson. HMSO, London.
6 Department of Health (1999) *Saving Lives: our healthier nation.* The Stationery Office, London.
7 Department of Health (1988) *Partnership in Action: new opportunities for joint working between health and social services.* HMSO, London.
8 Faculty of Public Health Medicine (2000) *Good Public Health Practice.* Royal College of Physicians, London.
9 Muir Gray J (1995) Is it worth doing? *Bandolier.* **1**: 2.

CHAPTER 9

Public participation in planning and delivering primary healthcare

Ruth Chambers

Public participation will not be effective unless we as health professionals and managers welcome the contribution that the public and patients can make to decision making. If public participation is to be meaningful we need to be ready and willing to listen to the public's informed views and shift power and resources accordingly.

The stages of public participation

The terms 'participation', 'consultation' and 'involvement' tend to be used interchangeably in popular parlance in the NHS. But 'participation' is used by others outside the NHS as the umbrella term that encompasses the progressively more participatory stages[1] of:

- information exchange: we give the public information, they give us information but we do not negotiate or develop a shared view
- consultation: the public and patients express their views but the consultant (a representative of the NHS in this case) makes decisions about developments
- support: the public decides what to do and others support them in doing it
- deciding together: thinking and planning together
- acting together: putting plans into action together.

'Involvement' is a rather vague term that is used to imply that some activity happened that brought the public or individual patients into contact with those working in the NHS to hear or receive views or information on a particular matter.

There are good examples of those working in primary care seeking patients' or the public's views, although the NHS does not have a tradition of doing so in a meaningful way. Those undertaking medical audit in primary care in the early 1990s sometimes included an element of public participation, usually at the first stage (see above) of information exchange. The focus of patient participation in medical audit was often on seeking users' views of the practice's services such as the comfort of the waiting room or ease of making appointments. Non-users' views were rarely sampled and the topics considered were usually relatively superficial, avoiding core aspects of the practice management or operation.

Patients' charters were another opportunity to seek patients' or the public's views in the 1990s, although the specified patients' rights and responsibilities expressed in patients' charters were usually drawn up unilaterally by the health service. Practices who adopted patients' charters often imposed 'off-the-peg' models on their patients rather than constructing charters in response to their patients' input.

Some general practices have experimented with patient participation groups but few of these have been used to provide informed views that are fed into strategic planning and development. Patient participation groups are of a wide range of types: they may be a mix between patient users or support groups, campaigning and advice groups, providers of social care and fundraisers. Members of patient participation groups may be invited or self-selected. Their objectives vary too and include: involving patients in planning services, co-ordinating volunteer programmes (for example, volunteer-run transport schemes for the elderly, visiting the practice or hospitals), developing health promotion and illness prevention, providing feedback on existing services, fundraising or a mix of these.

The culture of public participation in PCG and now PCT business has been very much shaped by the expectations of official documents emerging from the Department of Health over the last few years.[2–6] The import is to exhort those working in the NHS to 'promote patients' participation in their own care as active partners with professionals', to 'enable patients to become informed about their treatment and care and to make informed decisions and choices about it if they wish', to 'involve patients and carers in improving service quality' and to 'involve the public as citizens in health and health service decision making processes'.[5]

We should no longer be using 'public participation' as a means of bolstering decisions that have in reality already been taken. We should no longer be manipulating public opinion to justify NHS decisions that are based on one or two key people's preferences or historical patterns, as opposed to decisions made in response to fairly assessed need and rational debate.

The focus of public participation for PCTs as set out in Box 9.1 is to improve the health of the community. The community here includes users, carers, the local population, voluntary groups with an interest in health and non-health organisations such as local government departments (for example, education). The government expects the benefits to include:

> reductions in health inequalities, better outcomes of individual care, better health for the population, better quality and more locally responsive services, greater ownership of health services and a better understanding by all concerned of why and how local services need to be changed and developed.[6]

These expected benefits do seem a logical consequence of finding out and including people's views in decision making about health service developments so long as those consulted are well informed and comprehend all the issues, including resource constraints and the essential core business of the NHS.

Box 9.1   Improving the health of the community[7]

PCTs will take responsibility for improving the health of their community and addressing local health inequalities. They will need to ensure that a range of services are available for their population which are delivered to a consistently high quality and are efficient and effective. In meeting these requirements they will need to engage with and involve patients, carers and local partner organisations. The needs of their community might be met more effectively through partnership working or development and support of non-health service provision.

Information exchange

Information exchange is essential to the process of participation. A study by Dolan and colleagues[8] looked at how people rated priorities in healthcare before and after being given information and demonstrated how important it is for people to be well informed prior to being asked to make a decision about planning or delivering healthcare (Box 9.2).

Box 9.2   Effect of discussion and deliberation on the views of focus group participants

Sixty patients from two urban general practices in North Yorkshire each attended two focus group meetings, two weeks apart. About half of the participants initially wanted to give a lower priority to smokers, heavy drinkers and illicit drug users receiving healthcare, but by the end of the second meeting about one third of these no longer wanted to discriminate against such people. The participants' views about setting priorities in health-care were systematically different at the end of their second focus group meeting compared to the beginning of the first meeting, after they had been given opportunities to discuss the issues and had time for personal reflection.

Although public meetings inform the audience about the organiser's views of the issues, the attending audience cannot be said to be 'well informed' after such an event. Few of the public will have had the oppor-tunity or confidence to ask questions; those on the platform probably have entrenched beliefs and it is difficult for those listening to know whether they are being fed biased or balanced views of the issues, what the options are and what are the implications of alternative decisions.

Some PCGs have tried to make public meetings more meaningful by including talks by invited experts on, for example, clinical conditions such as mental health, diabetes or coronary heart disease. But any PCG/Ts who think that they are leading on public participation because they have attracted good numbers of the public to attend such events are mistaken as these mainly passive meetings are not the basis of true participation, which requires meaningful exchange of well-informed views between the public and health 'bosses' which leads to shared decision making.

A challenge for PCTs is to find meaningful ways to inform the public before asking them to participate in making decisions about healthcare issues. We are still at a very early stage in developing expertise in the NHS in knowing how best to inform the public in general and patients as individuals to enable them to participate in consultation exercises and contribute to decision making. We need to develop best practice in:

- the quality of information given to the public as part of the participa-tion process
- the quantity of information: depth, how many new concepts, is it appropriate for those receiving it?

- the mode of information giving: written, spoken, video, computer interactive, group work, postal documents – what works best and when?
- the setting for information exchange: neutral territory, public's home base
- involving experts: at what stage in the proceedings, who should select the experts, should the public and/or health professionals question the experts?
- involving professionals: at what stage in the proceedings, should professionals and managers mix in with the public or be brought in early/late in the process?
- avoiding bias in the information-giving process so that the public and individuals participating receive a balance of views from experts and interested parties.

Methods of information exchange and consultation

Some health authorities and local government departments have set up 'citizens' juries' and other types of 'health panels' to try to inform as well as consult their public. A typical citizens' jury has 10–20 people; jurors discuss and debate the issue in the light of written and verbal evidence from witnesses and experts before deciding on their verdict. Biases may be introduced by the way that the question is set for the jury to consider, the nature of the information and evidence presented to the jurors and the identities of the witnesses, interested parties and stakeholders who attend. An independent facilitator helps the process along. Jurors may be asked to choose between options drawn up by the organisers or to develop criteria to guide decisions on a particular issue. Jurors are not elected by the local population but recruited by independent organisations such as market research companies; they should reflect the profile of the population in question with respect to age, gender, employment status, ethnicity and geographical spread.

The outcomes of citizens' juries have varied from instances where the jury's report has influenced local decision making to examples where the jury's verdict coincided with other people's earlier recommendations which then took on a higher priority. Citizens' juries are costly to set up and run: typical costs are quoted as being around £16 000 plus considerable staff time, up to £30 000.[9]

Methods of recruitment to local health panels vary. Some are set up by advertising through the local press and media with the panel members further selected from these volunteers on the basis of their age, sex, ethnicity and relatively recent experiences of the NHS. Panel numbers range between 200 and 600 in different instances; some operate only by postal surveys whilst in others, additional focus groups are held in parallel with other survey work to allow more interactivity and exchange of information between organisers and panel members. Most health panels retain members for up to three years before replacing them.

Neighbourhood forums are another method of public participation where the organisers attempt to inform forum members about the issues by allowing opportunities for questions and increased understanding of the issues and supplying experts as requested by the forum, before views are formulated by forum members. Nineteen neighbourhood forums have been running in North Staffordshire for several years; members change regularly and include a mix of key or interested people in the locality, such as the clergy, nurses, teachers, etc.

Consultation

To consult the public means knowing who they are, why you are consulting them and how to select the most appropriate method for reaching and engaging with a particular subgroup of the population to whom the consultation relates. A meaningful consultation is one in which you exchange information and obtain a representative opinion that feeds into the local decision making process of your PCT and/or the participating practices.

Essential facets of meaningful consultation

Be clear about:

- the purpose of the exercise: is it important and is it necessary?
- the type and identity of the population to whom the purpose relates
- how to reach and engage the target population
- the extent and mode of information exchange required prior to consultation
- the implications of the methods you employ in the consultation: what biases will arise, is the expense of the consultation likely to be worthwhile?
- what outputs you expect from the consultation
- how you will act on the results of the consultation

- how you will feed back results to those who were consulted and the public in general
- how you will evaluate the consultation and rest of the public participation process.

The costs of the consultation may be considerable and you may have to trade off a relatively cheaper method of consultation that engages with fewer people or with a less representative section of the population subgroup than you would have ideally liked. The results of consulting the public about the same question in different arenas will vary according to the characteristics of the sample of the public questioned, the extent of prior information individuals already have and receive about the topic, and the mode of consultation.

Just as in any scientific exercise, it is important to know the implications of the methods that you choose so that you can make adjustments for any biases that arise from your limited consultation. You might try to reduce the effects of such biases by undertaking various methods of consultation around the same purpose so that your final picture is made up of several different inputs. You will have to decide whether in minimising resources spent on consultation, the effort will still be worthwhile and that the exercise is not merely a token gesture of consultation.

In formulating the NHS plan the government undertook a consultation exercise in the spring of 2000. This involved a mix of consultation methods including selective interviews and public meetings around the country, six working groups of key opinion leaders and a questionnaire for the general public: 12 million leaflets with prepaid response forms were distributed widely at public venues asking 'What are the top three things you think would make the NHS better for you and your family?'. The good response to the questionnaire survey of around a quarter of a million respondents demonstrates the public's enthusiasm for being involved in planning and developing the NHS.

The government's approach has been widely criticised for breaching best practice in consultation methodology,[11] particularly as the questionnaire method is unlikely to have attracted much response from already unrepresented minority groups (for example, those who do not speak English or young people). Nevertheless, the government now has a wealth of current views from this and previous consultation exercises, such as the previous national survey in 1999, on which to undertake more detailed consultative work.

A standing health panel with integral focus group or interviewing options may be a relatively low-cost method of consulting that also provides a meaningful response from the public, providing that the panel is set up to reflect a cross-section of the local population, the panel members are consulted in ways that allow everyone to contribute and the organiser presents panel members with sufficient balanced information to enable them to give an informed opinion. Care needs to be taken to include young and elderly groups who are often left out of consultation processes because they are more difficult to reach and engage or because travel difficulties, and physical and sensory limitations preclude them from attending meetings or completing questionnaires.

A challenge for PCTs in undertaking effective public consultation

Those working in the NHS are still at an early stage in understanding how to undertake consultation that is meaningful, affordable and worthwhile. The following challenges face PCTs:

- to understand the extent to which different methods of public consultation generate the same outputs and make allowances for this in the interpretation of the results of consultation
- to determine what modes of consultation are most likely to obtain meaningful views from different subgroups of the population
- to understand the characteristics of a public consultation process that predict the use of the results in the decision making process in the planning and delivery of healthcare
- how best to inform a representative section of the general population about issues that affect the general community or a subgroup of the population but do not normally affect them
- who should undertake the consultation: should it be the PCT or the health authority or should they employ an independent party? Who should plan the range of methods to be used?
- how PCTs can get a balance between expending resources consulting the majority of the population who are relatively easy to reach such as householders and minority subgroups who are relatively more difficult to reach but whose needs may be overlooked if they are not consulted
- how to bring constituent practices and general practice teams along with the culture of public participation, so that they share ownership of the decisions emerging from any public participation exercises arranged by their PCT's board
- how and to what extent lay members of PCT boards (just as lay members of PCG boards) should represent their local constituents' views, especially if they conflict with their own personally held opinions.

Supporting, deciding together, acting together

Community development provides opportunities for communities to recognise and meet their own needs, whilst working in partnership to influence service and strategic development,[1] as the example given in Box 9.3 shows. Community development tends to be targeted at people who are excluded from society or who share a common characteristic, such as being a young single parent or living on the same housing estate. Community development aims to help people 'tackle for themselves the problems which they face and identify to be important and empower them to change things by developing their own skills, knowledge and experience and by working in partnership with other groups and with statutory agencies'.[9] Focus groups, interviewing and observation inform the developmental work and the evaluation.

Box 9.3   Community participation in PCGs and the HAZ in Tyne and Wear[10]

The Newcastle Health Partnership has a strategy for city-wide community participation that aims to help local communities act on their own health agendas. Special efforts have been made to include black and ethnic minorities, gay and lesbian groups, older people, adolescents and people with a physical or sensory disability.

Health priorities emerged from the 90 local groups involved in the initiative and were taken up by health services management. The community worker and two lay members of the health action group have places on the local PCG's board. An annual local health conference is attended by more than 200 local people and develops priorities for the year's proposed health commissioning. They have found that public involvement leads to the NHS having a greater understanding of local health issues and new ways of tackling them. The two-way dialogue improves relationships and gives the public an insight into the pressures on health services too.

The stages of community development[1,9] are:

* analysis of community needs
* action planning towards solutions by local residents
* community priorities are turned into clear and measurable objectives for monitoring, evaluation and review

- adaptation and design of services in response to community's objectives and their input into strategic development.

Community development can provide the interface where the views from the public and individuals in their own settings, with their 'bottom-up' priorities, meet the 'top-down' priorities from the PCT board and other NHS origins to establish a forum where conflicting priorities, misunderstandings and misinformation can be resolved and shared decision making can happen.

Practical ways forward with public participation

Establish a health forum where issues and strategy concerning key issues can be debated

It is well known that the opinions of the public, patients who are intimately concerned with the issue (for example, the sufferer of the clinical condition in question), healthcare professionals and insurers differ.[12] Involving as many interested parties as possible in the health forum should make it less likely that the outcomes of work and participation exercises commissioned by the health forum will be marginalised and omitted from subsequent decision making at a strategic level.

Provide education and training for as many and as wide a cross-section of self-employed practitioners and employed staff working in your PCT as possible

Not only will many more learn the skills of undertaking the different stages of public participation and the methods of consultation such as focus groups, surveys and consensus exercises, but also the learners will be more aware of the benefits and limitations of public participation. Health visitors and other community nurses may be real assets in sharing their knowledge and experience of different stages in the process of public participation with others in the NHS workforce; local community development workers might similarly help train others less experienced in engaging with the local population.

Build up a network of all who are interested or active in public participation within your PCT area and across the district

You might construct shared databases of information and open access to your own sources of data, improving the extent of assessment of the population's health needs. Sharing ideas and resources should reduce duplication of effort by the professionals and consultation fatigue from the public's perspective. You might set up a community-wide intranet where health and non-health organisations can tap into a shared and established system for all stages of public participation from information giving to consultation to decision making to evaluation.

Focus on population subgroups that are relevant to the characteristics and health priorities of your resident population

These might include carers, the homeless, those with learning disability, or teenage parents, for example. You might encourage your constituent practices to help to identify individuals in these particular groups of people and with their permission enter their names on a database which can be used by others to target care and services at them.

Work at establishing a culture where public participation is welcomed and the advantages are recognised

The PCT board is likely to be far more enthusiastic and knowledgeable about methods of public participation and the benefits than others working in their constituent practices. The PCT board should support lay members in developing public and community involvement and participation within the PCT's constituency. You need to bring everyone along with you if public participation is to work out in practice so that will mean a systematic effort to explain why, what and how you are establishing public participation and disseminating news of the outcomes, showing when benefits have arisen that are unlikely to have occurred without public participation.

The PCT will know that it has succeeded when:

- meaningful public participation is an essential feature of any decision making about planning or development of all significant work in the PCT
- the PCT can demonstrate how the public's views were incorporated in finding ways to make the best use of limited resources.[13]

It will take time to convince not only your constituent practices but your local community that it is worth participating and to establish the conditions and know-how to actually do it.

References

1 Taylor M (1995) *Unleashing the Potential: bringing residents to the centre of regeneration*. Joseph Rowntree Foundation, York.
2 NHS Executive (1996) *Patient Partnership: building a collaborative strategy*. Department of Health, Leeds.
3 NHS Executive (1997) *The New NHS: modern, dependable*. Department of Health, London.
4 NHS Executive (1999) *Patient and Public Involvement in the New NHS*. Department of Health, Leeds.
5 Stuart G (1999) Government wants patient partnership to be integral part of NHS. *BMJ*. **319**: 788 (letter).
6 Department of Health (2000) *Interim Reports of the Six Modernisation Teams*. Confidential working documents. Department of Health, London.
7 Department of Health (1999) *Primary Care Groups: taking the next steps*. Associated documentation: *Primary Care Trusts: establishment, the preparatory period and their Functions*. HSC 1999/246: LAC (99) 40. Department of Health, London.
8 Dolan P, Cookson R and Ferguson B (1999) Effect of discussion and deliberation on the public's views of priority setting in health care: focus group study. *BMJ*. **318**: 916–19.
9 Chambers R (1999) *Involving Patients and the Public: how to do it better*. Radcliffe Medical Press, Oxford.
10 Crowley P and Freake D (1999) Reaping the rewards. PCG partners

the public. *Doctor.* **8 April:** 62–3.
11 Anderson W and Florin D (2000) Consulting the public about the NHS. *BMJ.* **320**: 153–4.
12 Stronks K, Strijbis AM, Wendte J *et al.* (1997) Who should decide? Qualitative analysis of panel data from public, patients, healthcare professionals, and insurers on priorities in health care. *BMJ.* **315**: 92– 6.
13 Audit Commission (2000) *The PCG Agenda.* Audit Commission, London.

Further reading

Barker J, Bullen M and de Ville J (1999) *Reference Manual for Public Involvement* (2e). South Thames Regional Office, NHS Executive, London.
Jordan J, Dowswell T, Harrison S *et al.* (1998) Whose priorities? Listening to users and the public. *BMJ.* **316**: 1668–70.
Ling T (ed.) (1999) *Reforming Healthcare by Consent.* Radcliffe Medical Press, Oxford.
NHS Executive (1999) *Public Engagement Toolkit.* Northern and Yorkshire Regional Office, NHS Executive, Durham.
Novartis (1999) *Engaging the Public Toolkit.* Novartis Pharmaceuticals, Richmond.

CHAPTER 10

IM&T for PCTs

Peter Smith

IM&T used effectively promises to revolutionise the understanding of health and the delivery of healthcare. It also threatens to become a white elephant that bestrides the NHS like a Colossus, depositing its ordure on those below. This will particularly be the case if developments are technology-led rather than driven by information needs.

Many apparently Everest-sized problems, such as primary care data, have recently begun to look more like manageable foothills, if not molehills. However, for PCTs straddling primary and community care, significant changes in IT infrastructure may be required to implement a vision that fully exploits the skills in primary care as part of systems of integrated care. The vision was laid out in *Information for Health*,[1] the first really comprehensive blueprint for an IT-rich NHS.

Many PCGs have had to tolerate data voids as they have struggled to get to grips with organisational issues. PCTs cannot afford the luxury. Their unique position as purchaser and provider demands comprehensive and exhaustive knowledge of their own and others' performance. For PCTs, deficiencies in data can prevent the best laid of plans from reaching fruition.

There must be no data 'no-go areas' where the data 'isn't very good', whether in primary or secondary care. PCTs must demand and deliver good data. Primary care is relatively cheap, secondary care is not. The resource associated with a small 'variation in the accuracy' of a trust's data would be enough to pay for a significant primary care development.

Feedback of information based on the PCTs' data is vital if changes are sought and if PCTs and their practices are to understand the relevance and importance of data collection. Only then will the need for accurate recording be fully accepted.

Having been involved in the production of the January 2000 IM&T guidance,[2] I have drawn heavily upon its principles in this chapter. It contains extensive extra advice and I can fully recommend it. It is available on the Department of Health website.[3]

Planning services

PCTs should take a full and active part in determining the priorities, targets and use of resources within the Local Implementation Strategy (LIS). Hopefully, most PCGs moving to PCT status will have been fully involved with the LIS process to ensure that allocation of resources supports their PCT aspirations. For instance, if the LIS has tied up most existing funding, they may find they have restricted capability for developing new systems at PCT and practice level. PCT IM&T development will need to be flagged up early in the LIS process.

Successful implementation of the information strategy relies upon specialist informatics functions. The informatics skills of current information departments at trust and HA level will need to be used effectively, co-ordinating the use of existing information within the health community.

IM&T in primary care

Using clinical data

PCTs will need to use data in primary care clinical systems to support planning, commissioning, monitoring and evaluation of services. For example:

- establishing prevalence of disease, including changes
- monitoring activity (contacts, interventions, referrals)
- movements towards health targets
- chronic diseases treatment protocols
- outcomes for patients with specified illness
- targeting at-risk groups
- supporting clinical governance
- clinical audit
- benchmarking using comparative data between practices in a PCT
- assessing the impact of primary care developments and integration
- changing service provision.

A senior professional should take responsibility for planning and implementing agreed actions to assess and improve primary care data quality, and to analyse and make use of the data as outlined above.

Both a GP lead and/or data quality facilitator will be needed to focus on this work at PCT level.

Breaking down data barriers

Current practice systems have of necessity been GP focused. Successive Requirements for Accreditation (RFAs) have correctly insisted upon this. However, their use can be extended to facilitate integration.

Level 4 PCTs in particular should consider strategies for moving towards systems that are used by both primary care and community care services. The development of a shared electronic patient record will be the key to development of many services.

Clinical systems will continue to operate at the level of the individual practice, as now. Communications links and data exchanges between them will assist integration. Many of the benefits of integration can still be achieved with the current fragmented and patchy system. Caldicott[4] issues (see below) will be paramount, including definition of the 'need to know' for different levels of access to the electronic patient record.

A programme that moves towards integration could include:

- introducing extra terminals with suitable data entry templates to practice systems for the use of community nurses and midwives
- undertaking a training programme
- defining local Read codes where the system permits (e.g. the Torex Meditel 6000 system that allows user-defined Read codes that might include purely health visitor functions)
- local standards for recording community nursing activities on practice systems, minimising multiple data entry.

Any process must have clinical support and be phased, taking account of the legal status of GP clinical records, consistency of use and coding, training and resources determined by the LIS process.

Where NHS community trusts already use patient-centred systems, PCTs may want to retain them, though they will require good electronic exchange of information with practices to make best use of the information. Good interchange will facilitate the clinical process, as well as assist in planning and delivering the data requirements of the NSFs.

Data quality

Easily accessible, good-quality information obtained from routinely entered data is essential to any programme of improvement in primary care but use of practice clinical systems is at best variable, at worst chaotic. The legal necessity for practices to retain a paper record will continue to hamper the move to a full electronic patient record. Legitimisation of the electronic patient record is long overdue.

Migration to electronic records may take several years and will require training and financial support. Meanwhile, an approach that encourages 'information maturity' could be usefully adopted. Such a scheme would increase the usage and coverage of clinical recording within practice systems. It can only work if the effort is put in at practice and professional level. Management of the process by PCT edict will be doomed to failure.

PCTs will need to:

- assess the level of information maturity of their constituent practices
- develop the use, coverage and accuracy of clinical recording.

Simple, really!

Fortunately, there should be little need to create new wheels. Some pretty robust ones are already available: the GPIMM and the CHDGP project.

GPIMM

The General Practice Information Maturity Model is well described in *Information and IT for Primary Care.*[5] It covers six levels of maturity, analysing several aspects of IM&T use (Table 10.1).

Table 10.1 The six levels of the GPIMM

Level	Designation	Summary description
0	Paper based	The practice has no computer system
1	Computerised	The practice has a computer system used only by practice staff
2	Computerised PHC team	The practice has a computer system used by practice staff and the PHC team, including doctors
3	Coded	The system makes limited use of Read codes
4	Bespoke	The system is tailored to the needs of the practice through agreed coding policies and the use of clinical protocols
5	Paperless	The practice is completely paperless, except where paper records are a legal requirement

My own favoured term for the final group is 'IT rich'. 'Paperless' is perhaps still something of a misnomer until all NHS records are IT-based; witness the piles of paper that greet the visitor to a paperless practice. Also, paperless has often meant 'information free' as systems are inadequately developed.

GPIMM can be administered by a simple piece of software obtainable from Alan Gillies (see Appendix 2 in reference[5]). It also includes advice on priorities according to the data entered, which covers:

- computerisation
- personnel usage
- coding
- system usage
- electronic patient records.

Having established an IT baseline, the next step is to look at developing the entry and use of accurate data.

CHDGP project

The Collection of Health Data in General Practice project developed a detailed, practical model for the recording and use of accurate data in general practice. As of April 2000, it has been administered by PRIMIS (Primary Care Information Services), based in Nottingham.[6] The system developed by CHDGP includes everything from detailed instructions for facilitators to standardised Read codes (yes, it's already been done!) covering the six areas:

- heart disease and related conditions
- cerebrovascular disease and related conditions
- hypertension
- diabetes
- asthma
- severe mental illness.

Two extremely useful manuals are available from the NHSIA website completely free. They are:

- *CDHGP Guidelines*, including many areas presented as 'fact sheets' for general distribution.[7]
- *Facilitators Handbook*, giving detailed instructions on every practical aspect of implementing a data quality improvement scheme.[8]

Despite significant criticism, the use of MIQUEST to interrogate systems and amalgamate useful data is likely to be the NHS standard. The CHDGP project made sole use of MIQUEST for interrogating systems and detailed instructions on its uses are included.

Both documents are obtainable from the NHSIA website at http://www.nhsia.nhs.uk

Clinical terms

Read coding is the standard system of coding used in general practice. This is to be amalgamated with the system used by the College of American Pathologists (CAP), SNOMED RT, to create a new clinical language system, called SNOMED Clinical Terms. This will be available from late 2001.

Prescribing

Currently, each GP practice is allocated an indicative prescribing budget. PMS pilots may be allocated a real budget (at the time of writing the author's practice was one of only two or three PMS pilots that had taken this up). PCTs will continue to have the responsibility of monitoring and influencing the prescribing behaviour of GPs in their area. All PCGs are currently required to operate prescribing incentive schemes. This is likely to be the case with PCTs.

Prescribing of practices within PCTs will be monitored by the PCT, not the HA. Therefore prescribing data for such practices will be in the domain of the PCT. HAs will only require aggregate figures at PCT level.

The Prescription Pricing Authority (PPA) provides PCTs with electronic prescribing systems and paper reports to support monitoring of prescribing. This is either in the form of paper reports or in electronic (EPACT) form.

PCT prescribing cost statements are now available showing monthly cumulative expenditure and forecast expenditure, as well as at practice level. Costs should continue to be attributed to 'the most relevant cost centre', usually the GP practice.

Prescribing Analyses and Cost (PACT) and the Prescribing Toolkit
EPACT (electronic PACT) is available online. It allows authorised officers in a PCT to access information on their constituent practices.

The Prescribing Toolkit system provides for the analysis of constituent practice data according to many criteria, including generic use and potential savings and against several prescribing indicators validated by the NHSE Prescribing Indicators Group (rather self-deprecatingly termed PIG).

Combining the use of this prescribing analysis with clinical data will provide a powerful tool for both clinical governance and HImPs.

GPNet/ Project Connect

The GPNet initiative is refocused on delivering networked clinical applications to primary care professionals' desktops (rather than just to practices) by the use of local area networks (LANs).

As a result, the GPNet programme has been re-scoped and further information is now available: see http://www.gpnet.nhsia.nhs.uk

PCT feedback

There is good evidence that feedback can be a potent means of changing behaviour. It also confirms to practices that the information they have been spending their precious time on is actually being analysed. Guidance has already required the introduction of prescribing and HCHS incentive schemes, with the January 2000 guidance referring to practices as 'cost centres'. Whatever one's beliefs, until practices and PHCTs feel included in the process, there will be limited opportunities to make significant changes.

Modern IM&T offers the opportunity to provide feedback that encourages PHCTs and practices to look at their activity in a non-threatening fashion. Once the efficient collection of data at practice level is achieved, whether through incentives or otherwise, there is the real possibility that systems can be developed to include educational support. At such a point, IT, clinical governance, education and data collection combine to produce a powerful driver of change and improvements in practice.

IM&T Supporting Commissioning

Information on secondary and tertiary care

NHS-Wide Clearing System (NWCS) data

Data sets on NWCS include well over 100 fields and should be available on at least a monthly basis. In practice, the data may well be several months out of date. Trusts should be required to ensure the accuracy and completeness of data. These aspects should be covered in an information agreement. A prospective agreement might be introduced which sets penalties to be introduced into the round of agreements made in the subsequent year.

PCTs will require commissioning data sets identifiable at individual PCT and practice level.

PCTs should now receive regular monthly reports on admitted patients covered by service agreements. Some of the old problems of double accounting inherent in the old 'finished consultant episode' (FCE) have been ironed out by the use of 'spells' which cover the whole period of admission, although FCEs are still recorded. These should now include:

• records of FCEs and spells including day cases and inpatients
• identification by trust and by practice
• comparisons against previous year's data
• speciality level reports covering lengths of stay and comparisons against previous years for each trust.

PCTs will be able to 'drill down' beneath the data presented in the reports to look at practice, GP-specific and consultant-specific data. A record of GP and consultant codes may be required for identification.

Information relating to outpatient care

Currently it is not a mandatory requirement for NHS trusts to provide outpatient commissioning data sets to HAs via NWCS.

Patients using emergency services

It is not mandatory for trusts to provide information on A&E attendances, but it is clearly essential information for monitoring the effects of service changes such as walk-in centres, co-operatives, ICPs and local accident reduction targets.

PCTs may be able to come to local agreements on A&E data, starting perhaps with a download of relevant data to be analysed at PCT level.

Waiting lists

PCTs should provide regular, accurate data on waiting lists to individual practices. PCTs themselves should aggregate this data to establish monitor service agreements and long-term service agreements (LTSAs). This information must be up to date for effective monitoring of referrals, particularly when part of an agreed protocol.

Again, although not mandatory, PCTs should look to trusts to provide this information as part of a local information agreement. This will enable practices to 'validate' waiting lists and to notify NHS trusts of patients who:

• are no longer registered
• have died
• have already been treated
• no longer require treatment.

Funding of this validation process should be commensurate with the work involved.

Information agreements

The prime responsibility for ensuring the accuracy, consistency and comprehensiveness of clinical details within commissioning data sets lies with NHS trusts. Evidence suggests that secondary care data has become less accurate since the demise of the internal market. There is now less of an incentive to produce accurate data. Information agreements should start to address this problem by defining local data quality standards.

Agreements should cover commissioning and clinical data quality. Reciprocal agreements should cover information flows between NHS trusts, HAs, PCTs and individual practices. Methods for monitoring the agreements by at least sample validation will need to be agreed.

Confidentiality and access issues (see below under 'Caldicott issues') should be addressed in detail and agreed between the relevant Caldicott guardians (see below).

Integrated care pathways (ICPs)

ICPs are particularly valuable for patients with chronic conditions where care is delivered in various settings. For ICPs to work, data collection and analysis systems that support the use of modified community data sets will need to be set up. These may be replaced by HRG developments in the near future. To fully inform the ICP process, information is required from all types of provider covering all aspects of care delivered within a defined timescale.

Information required will be:

• problem
• aim of care
• care provider
• interventions/activities
• setting in which care was provided
• resources used
• outcomes of care.

Such collection and analysis is unlikely to be possible with most systems currently in use. In fact, much of this information may just not be available and may be difficult to obtain in any sort of reliable form for some time. However, these community data sets are the gold standard requirement for future services development. PCTs will need to develop a capability that supports this if they are to adequately analyse care delivered in different settings and ultimately to deliver effective integrated care. HRG developments in the offing may provide some of the solutions to these issues.

From data to information for commissioning

Both service agreements and LTSAs will require data to be converted into useful information. Various analyses will be necessary to generate the building blocks for useful planning. This activity information may be:

• obtained and amalgamated form individual practice clinical systems
• commissioning data sets via the NWCS and received from NHS trusts
• obtained directly from trusts by local agreements or by accessing the trusts' databases directly.

Value added

Data will require manipulation and analysis to be turned into worthwhile information. Examples could be:

- *referrals*: comparisons of levels and patterns of referrals in year against historic data and between practices and for monitoring effects of new protocols (e.g. according to new NSFs)
- *activity*: within all sectors of the local health economy to formulate LTSAs and monitor them
- *indicators and benchmarks:* for process and outcomes indicative of good practice, compliance with agreements, indicators of access and efficiency. Dealing with inequalities will be a major aim.

LTSAs will be based on particular conditions. The analyses above will need to be able to indicate difference across different populations and between practices within the PCT area. Analysis by HRG and using national cost reference comparisons will be essential.

To support the analysis above, the following will need to be established:

- change in need and demand over time
- access to services: rates for various different local and practice populations
- patient pathway analyses from presentation through referral, assessment and diagnosis, treatment and discharge. To monitor holistic quality of ICPs agreed within LTSAs.

Systems support for information management and analysis

One single system is unlikely to deliver all the requirements for information management. However, flexible open-ended solutions could be created by amalgamating data from clinical systems and commissioning data sets. Increasingly, data will need to be stored in 'data repositories'.

At a very simple level these could be within Excel spreadsheets. Information from the NWCS can be downloaded into Excel and manipulated. However, use of databases with integrated management tools provides a more powerful means of obtaining answers and presenting useful information. With staff capable of such feats in short supply, this is an area that cries out for the local informatics service described in *Information for Health*.

The Commissioning Toolkit
An NHSE Commissioning Toolkit, to be made available at the end of 2000, will allow comparisons of activity data between PCTs and providers. This will be potentially powerful software that will present

data in useful graphical fashion. The addition of costed HRGs will once again permit the detailed analysis of where the resource is being used and will prompt PCTs to ask searching questions of themselves and their providers.

It is hoped that similar software is to be made available to provide practice-level comparisons.

IM&T support for health needs assessment

PCTs will need to work closely with their local public health department, who will have extensive expertise in this area. They will need to analyse a wide range of information when assessing the health status and needs of their local populations and developing the services to meet them.

Data support health needs assessment can be obtained from a variety of sources and needs to include:

- age and sex profiles (obtained from Family Health Services (FHS) registers)
- area-based estimates and projections are produced by the Office of National Statistics (ONS)
- prevalence and incidence of diseases and problems which may be obtained from information derived from practice and other clinical systems, from local disease registers and from national data sets such as the public health data set and from birth and death registration data supplied by ONS
- population and household characteristics may be derived from ONS census data, local registers, local surveys and national market research surveys
- 'environmental' information.

Planning services

Activity and forecast analyses will need to be combined with financial and resource information to plan and monitor services. Information required will include:

- financial allocations including modernisation funds and budgets to establish current and forecast expenditure
- services capacities, including premises, available beds, staffing capacity and potential for service modification
- professional and managerial capacity (to ensure fit with service needs)

- service costs, including national reference cost schedules based on HRGs.

Comparative analysis of this information will be helpful, between practices, PCTs and with other populations. Benchmarking will help to provide understanding of variations.

Improving quality

Various quality initiatives form the backbone of the New NHS. Broadly, these are to drive up standards and reduce 'unacceptable' variations in service. They include clinical governance and National Service Frameworks (*see* below).

The National Institute for Clinical Excellence (NICE) and NSFs will define the standards. They will be delivered through service agreements, annual accountability agreements and clinical governance.

It is worth reiterating that PCTs will become reliant on good information. It is therefore in the interest of the PCT if all practices are provided with hardware, software and training to ensure the delivery of increasingly accurate data. This may mean 100% reimbursement for equipment with funding from several different sources (including LIS monies). Having put the kit and capability in place, PCTs will need to consider how to provide access to good information sources in convenient and timely fashion.

National Service Frameworks

National Service Frameworks set the national standards and define the service models through which the NHS will provide and monitor a modern, comprehensive service. The intention is to drive up quality and minimise inconsistencies across the NHS at primary, secondary and tertiary levels.

Information will be required at all levels to support the NSFs.

It is beyond the scope of this book to cover specific National Service Frameworks. The Coronary Heart Disease NSF alone covers around 414 pages.

Example: coronary heart disease (CHD)
The CHD NSF[9] specifies that GPs and PHCTs should identify everyone with recognised CHD, TIA, stroke and peripheral vascular disease and put in place a model of care that ensures good management. This secondary prevention timescale is short. The use of the surrogate

marker of nitrate prescriptions recorded in a practice database will identify the majority of patients with ischaemic heart disease (IHD).

Having achieved this, there is then a stipulation that primary prevention is addressed, including identification of risk factors.

In both these areas, all but the most sophisticated of IT-rich practices
will require assistance with implementation. MIQUEST could be used
supportively to help practices with feedback on progress.

Resources will be made available for specific aspects of the NSF. Put
simply, each PCT will have to be able to put together a case for access to
these extra monies.

Integration of care

The use of shared information between primary and secondary care will
assist the process of integration and will eventually provide a seamless
information flow. PCTs will also be expected to look seriously at closer
integration between health and social care. There are three aspects of
working together that will facilitate this process:

• sharing information
• sharing staff and other resources
• pooling budgets.

Sharing information

For integration to succeed, health and social services will have to share
patient/client information. Caldicott principles will need to be enshrined
within any agreement made on the use of patient-identifiable data.
Attitudes towards confidentiality often differ across the health/social
interface, so the issues need to be handled sensitively. Patient expectations also need to be considered. A patient might not want information
divulged to a GP to be accessible to Social Services or vice versa.
Discussions around Caldicott may help.

Very often, data can be shared by having systems 'side by side'. This
might mean access to Social Services databases via a single terminal. If
using ordinary phone lines, confidentiality will be a major consideration,
with encryption essential. Agreement with the PCT Caldicott guardian
will be required. Once NHSNet is fully enabled, sharing may be less problematic. At a practice level, clinical systems could be shared with social
care members of the team.

Sharing staff and other resources

The new flexibilities referred to below allow sharing of resources across the health/social care interface. Scarce informatics resources could be shared, as could staff training.

Once information entry and sharing have been agreed, with the new flexibilities it is possible that home care may be managed at the interface, in which case access to clinical systems may be appropriate.

Pooling budgets

Recently, flexibilities have been introduced to allow pooling of budgets across health and social care. This offers great opportunities to integrate services, particularly at the home care level. The issue of Social Services not being free at the point of delivery needs to be considered carefully.

Confidentiality and security

Caldicott issues

The Caldicott Committee recommended several principles covering a local framework of responsibility to safeguard and govern uses of patient-identifiable information.

The principles are:

- justify the purpose(s) for which patient-identifiable data is to be used
- don't use patient-identifiable information unless it is absolutely necessary
- use the minimum necessary patient-identifiable information
- access to patient-identifiable information should be on a strict need-to-know basis
- everyone with access to patient-identifiable information should be aware of their responsibilities
- understand and comply with the law.

Each PCT should nominate a 'Caldicott guardian' who will need to work closely with individual practices to ensure that they have their own appropriate policies and frameworks in place. This will require a comprehensive audit.

Practice-identifiable information

Most practices are used to receiving comparative data, but some are still reluctant to agree to their own data being available for scrutiny. Referral patterns and prescribing are areas that can usefully be analysed in this fashion. However, the issue needs to be handled sensitively and even if the practice has agreed to data being used, variations should be discussed with practices before being made available to a wider audience. The NHS has managed to retain a semblance of a blame-free culture. This is particularly important where NHS data is concerned. Accuracy may be questionable and a variety of confounding factors may operate.

For instance, a practice known to the author was 'accused' of referring large numbers of patients with mild mental illness to a community mental health team. Further analysis showed that the practice manages most of their seriously mentally ill patients in-practice with the support of the CPN. Because they rarely need the input of a psychiatrist, they are not classed as seriously mentally ill. Confusing classifications here produced a picture that was the opposite of the reality.

Management arrangements

Guidance recommends that a subcommittee of each PCT executive should be established, including the Caldicott guardian, to control all aspects of local usage of patient- or practice-specific data. This subcommittee should devise and agree a confidentiality policy covering all data encountered within the PCT and define who is to oversee its implementation and subsequent operation.

A confidentiality policy should define:

- who has access to what information
- for what reasons
- the uses to which the data will be put
- to whom the information may be divulged.

It will be necessary to access patient- and practice-identifiable data for validation, monitoring and quality issues. Only named operatives should be allowed access.

A useful document is available covering Caldicott issues.[10]

IM&T supporting the business of PCTs

Office and communications systems

There is a wealth of commercially available software covering office functions and communications. They can help to minimise management costs, improving efficiency and assisting with the openness required of a public service organisation.

Office systems can provide PCTs with:

- consistent document standards and electronic publishing of reports to minimise costs
- professional-looking newsletter capability (for both internal and external uses)
- database capabilities with attractive, readable reports.

Email offers fast and efficient delivery of the standardised documents referred to above, reducing the paperchase that bedevils the modern office. Document archives on email systems allow the depositing of documents for all to read at leisure and to refer back to. With the swift publishing of HSCs on the Department of Health website, traditional difficulties with access to the latest guidance can be minimised.

Email between practices and with trusts provides the opportunity for greater communication. Since most of these contacts will not be referring to patient-identifiable data, simple systems can be used until the NHSNet is fully functioning.

Financial management and monitoring at the 'four levels'

PCG baseline
It could be reasonably assumed that PCGs will already have in place systems (usually at HA level, for PCG use) for:

- managing and monitoring their unified allocations
- supporting commissioning and monitoring service agreements
- maintaining activity information
- establishing budgets covering service agreements with providers
- planning and monitoring of expenditure on service agreements and LTSAs
- scenario planning when examining the impact of proposed changes at

PCT and practice level
- managing practice-level indicative budgets in the context of commissioning and service agreement monitoring
- 'benchmarking' GMS cash-limited allocations at practice level.

For those that are in any doubt about the need for practice-level information, recent IM&T guidance[3] states:

> *This will require the analysis of individual practice budget and expenditure information against 'averages' for the whole PCT and HA. This analysis will need to take account of variations in the size of practices and in their patient profiles, and will need to be supported by information on staff group hours, premises and equipment.*

Level 3 and 4 PCTs

Primary care development
The responsibility invested in the freestanding PCT is significantly greater than for PCGs. It is also less predictable how such organisations will develop given the wide range of different local circumstances. All PCTs will have to develop novel ideas. Just demonstrating they can deliver the same services as well as their predecessors will not be sufficient. The greater level of flexibility and sensitivity resulting from their knowledge of primary care will need to be exploited to the full.

The primary care investment plan referred to in Chapter 4 will need to reflect the application of these management IT functions in supporting primary care developments. Such capability has never existed before and the potential for using it to support primary care and general practice in particular is exciting.

Financial management and monitoring
Both levels 3 and 4 PCTs will need to combine their activity monitoring systems and related database tools with financial management and monitoring systems that can separate their expenditure on commissioning and providing services.

PCGs of necessity used modified HA systems to support financial management and monitoring. PCTs have a different relationship with the HA and any agreement with the HA authority will need to reflect this. Until they have sufficient in-house skills, they should therefore either:

- consider using the system on a contract basis, with a separate PCT account set-up or

- commission the services from another NHS trust (the community trust with whom the PCT is associated).

The first of these options is the most appropriate for a level 3 PCT, the second for a level 4 PCT.

PCT level 4 issues

PCTs should consider with their practices how to provide information systems to support integrated PHCTs, including GPs, nurses and other community workers.

In addition, level 4 PCTs will deliver community services. Most will be providing community nursing services, but some may deliver services in a community hospital setting. The role of level 4 PCTs in employing staff to provide health services will necessitate the development of an in-house system to cost services and manage service budgets and expenditure.

As service providers, PCTs will have additional needs and responsibilities.

- In line with their primary care development responsibilities, level 4 PCTs will have to have systems that can identify service and expenditure budgets at practice level.
- As part of their wider responsibilities, their systems will have to support the identification of data for national reference cost purposes.
- Where there are PMS pilots in the PCT area, separate accounts will need to be identified.
- Separate agreement and monitoring processes will be needed where they provide services outside the immediate PCT area.

Payroll systems

Most areas have achieved considerable efficiencies by local agency-type relationships covering payroll management and support. It would be a brave PCT that decided to change such arrangements.

Human resources and personnel systems

The NHS trust associated with the PCT is likely to have systems to manage these areas, including staff appraisal, development and professional development, nursing cover and the monitoring of sickness absences.

Existing trust systems are usually integrated with other systems, including payroll and clinical resource management systems that deal with sickness and maternity cover.

Setting up such systems *de novo* in the early stages would be unnecessarily time consuming, although it would need to be considered at some stage. Until then an agency arrangement would be appropriate.

Capital asset and equipment management

Management and maintenance of property and equipment will be the responsibility of level 4 PCTs. The scale of assets to be managed will depend on the range of services provided and will vary across PCTs.

As in the case of business systems, until the longer term requirements are clear and the necessary expertise is developed within the PCT, it will probably be preferable to make use of existing NHS trust systems on a 'bureau' basis.

In the early stages, where existing community trust systems are adequate, it is difficult to see how different aspects of these functions could be separated out for management of the IT function at PCT level. It is clearly for the PCT to decide on the meaning of the data and how it should be used creatively.

PCTs will need to establish how they can use this data to improve services in the new framework of the PCT; for example, to provide more seamless primary care services or clearer, costed ICPs straddling primary and secondary care.

Central information requirements

A PCT will have to supply data for central returns if it is responsible for or has had services delegated to it. It will also have to supply information to allow the HA to produce its Service and Financial Framework (SAFF) and associated returns to the Department of Health.

Where level 4 PCTs provide inpatient or day case treatments or care (e.g. elderly services), they must provide admitted patient care data sets to commissioning organisations via the NWCS.

The NHS Executive will not routinely monitor PCT activity. HAs will performance manage PCTs and regional offices of the NHSE will performance manage HAs.

Conclusion

This chapter merely scratches the surface of IM&T issues for PCTs. The NHS Plan suggests many new initiatives, on top of the many begun under the aegis of *Information for Health*. The rapid change will render large parts of this chapter obsolete by the time it is published. Despite the pace of change, PCTs cannot afford to fall behind, particularly on the IM side.

To quote General Patten: 'It is better that we act upon our imperfect plan today. We could perfect it within a week, but by that time we will have been overrun.'

References

1 NHS Executive (1998) *Information for Health*. HMSO, London.
2 NHS Executive (2000) *IM & T Requirements to Support PCGs and PCTs*. HMSO, London and online as in ref[3].
3 http://www.doh.gov.uk/nhsexipu/whatnew/pcguide.pdf
4 Caldicott Committee (1997) *Report on the Review of Patient Identifiable Information*. Department of Health, London.
5 Gillies A (1999) *Information and IT for Primary Care*. Radcliffe Medical Press, Oxford.
6 http://www.primis.nottingham.ac.uk/
7 http://www.nottingham.ac.uk/chdgp/guidelin.htm
8 http://www.nottingham.ac.uk/chdgp/handbook.htm
9 Department of Health (2000) *National Service Framework for Coronary Heart Disease*. HMSO, London
10 NHS Executive (2000) *Protecting and Using Patient Information: a manual for Caldicott guardians*. HMSO, London and: http://www.doh.gov.uk/confiden/cgmcont.htm

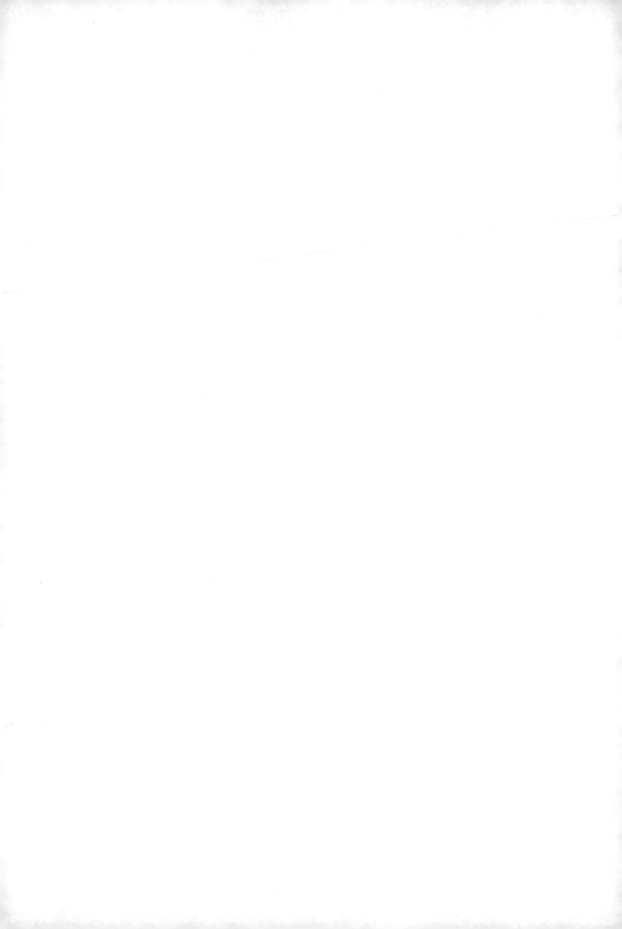

CHAPTER 11

Primary care franchises: a contractual alternative

John Oldham

The issues concerning the independent status of GPs are often surrounded by polemic. This is usually embedded in a particular and polarised political philosophy. The advocates of a salaried service will argue that general practice should be on the same basis as every other part of the NHS and clinically managed as such. On the other hand, equally vociferous supporters of independence regard it as a bastion of professional status and, looking at their consultant colleagues, fear the consequences of such change.

Which is right? Certainly there are more younger GP's wishing for salaried service, principally as a bulwark against out-of-hours work and the burden of equity purchase. There could also be a perception that one outcome of policy movement may be towards that end. However, just as we should utilise best-evidenced practice, so we should operate under the canopy of best evidence of management.

First principles of organisational design and behaviour teach us that form should follow function. The operating environment within which an organisation exists is key to the form which it should take to maximise harmony with the team. Key factors that mould structure are environmental complexity and uncertainty. Briefly, the more stable an environment, the more rigid can be the structure, with a list of rigid policies relatively unchanging. The more turbulent an environment, the greater is the need to ensure flexibility in the way people operate. The NHS is not a homogeneous organism with equivalent environmental determinants throughout it. One size cannot fit all.

The operating environment of primary care is one of rapidly changing technology and medical techniques, pressure on resources, changing data requirements, changing reputations, changing organisational relationships, shifting patient needs and demands because of demographic and social trends, and changing epidemiology and sporadic epidemics. Primary care has to cope with these factors as well as being vulnerable, as any service organisation, to demographic changes affecting labour availability. In addition, general practice faces competitive threats because of the lowering of barriers for other organisations to deliver aspects of primary care. In short, what might have been considered a complex, though stable, environment is a complex and unstable one.

Theory (and practice) maintains that an organisation will function best if its social and technical systems (tools, procedures, skills) are designed to optimise the demands of each other and the environment. For primary care, flat, flexible, devolved structures with short management decision loops are the best fit.

By default or design, this is what independent contractor status with practice-employed staff has given us. Yet clearly all is not well. The independence that has permitted innovation and successful adaptation in most places has allowed isolationism and poor practice elsewhere. Clearly it must be a policy goal that the level of service a patient experiences walking into any NHS provider, including primary care, is of an equivalent high standard. The reflex answer of exerting control by subsuming practices into a large organisation subject to line management and hierarchical decision making ill fits the requirement of the operating environment of primary care.

Similarly, continuation of the existing system of independent contractorship without greater accountability for quality is not an option. Clinical governance will clearly affect this equation positively but there is, to coin a phrase, a third way – franchise arrangement. The national GP contract is acknowledged by an increasing body of opinion to be outdated for a modern NHS. PMS pilots have demonstrated a variation on the theme. PMS also allows much greater flexibility in the personnel and skill mix within a primary care team, which itself reflects on the variety of services offered to patients. It also provides the means of greater accountability, whilst preserving the key features of primary care essential to the flexibility alluded to, including independent contractor status.

Franchises: what they might be and how they might operate

A NHS franchise in primary care could be a fixed term contract (five years) to offer primary care to a defined population under terms agreed locally with a health authority or PCT operated via a PMS contract. It is vital that the detailed terms of the contract should be locally determined to reflect the priorities and situation of the particular population, whilst reflecting the national goals of the NHS.

Each franchise would be subject to an annual review by the contracting authority. If the franchise had met the obligation of the contract at the end of the franchise period then the renewal for a further five years would be automatic.

If performance was below that expected at an annual review then the following might occur.

Correction is encouraged and the situation reviewed six months later. If concern existed at the third annual review and persisted at the fourth, then the franchisee would be informed that if correction had not occurred during the following six months, the franchise would be either:

- renewed on a reduced term with firm performance measures or
- offered to other franchisees, the notice period for the franchise being the final six months.

During that six months, other franchisees would be invited to operate the failing franchise. They may of course retain some or all personnel but have them working differently to their own proven protocols and systems.

A franchise system fits with rolling out clinical governance/NSFs and other measures of performance within a PCG/T. It also enables practices and practice teams to grow and progress even within more laggardly PCG/Ts. Efficiencies and improvements created by the franchises could reflect directly in their own organisation and its care delivery. This incentive would itself encourage improvement.

Attention to motivation is important in the functioning of any organisation. Poorly motivated individuals will work below their effective level of performance and may influence others and demotivate them. Management literature exposes several factors related to job design which stimulate intrinsic motivation: meaningfulness, responsibility, degree of autonomy and knowledge of results. Absence of one or more of these factors was shown to be demotivating. Franchise systems would ensure that in current organisational change these motivating factors were maintained for general practice.

Index

As the book is concerned with Primary Care Trusts only minimal use of this term and its acronym has been made in the index.